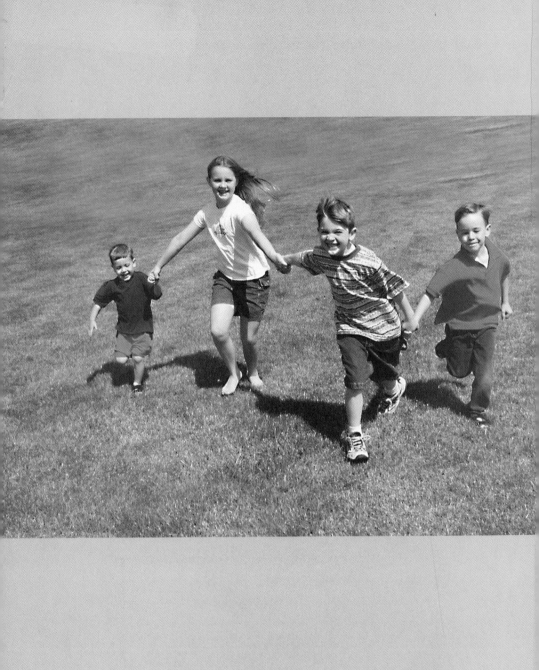

Camping with Kids

By Goldie Gendler Silverman

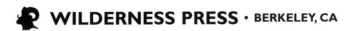
WILDERNESS PRESS · BERKELEY, CA

3812400059200

J
796.54
SILVER

Camping with Kids: The Complete Guide to Car, Tent, and RV Camping

1st EDITION January 2006

Copyright © 2006 by Goldie Gendler Silverman

Front cover photo copyright © 2006 by Mike Calabro, www.urbancamper.com
Back cover photo copyright © 2006 by Mike Calabro
Interior photos credited on page 252
Illustrations copyright © 2006 by Sarah Silverman
Cover and book design: Lisa Pletka
Book editor: Eva Dienel

ISBN 0-89997-361-2
UPC 7-19609-97361-4

Manufactured in the United States of America

Published by: **Wilderness Press
1200 5th Street
Berkeley, CA 94710
(800) 443-7227; FAX (510) 558-1696
info@wildernesspress.com
www.wildernesspress.com**
Visit our website for a complete listing of our books and for ordering information.

Cover photos:	Father, daughter, sitting by campfire *(front)*
	Boy with marshmallow *(back)*
Frontispiece:	Happy children running

All rights reserved. No part of this book may be reproduced in any form, or by any means electronic, mechanical, recording, or otherwise, without written permission from the publisher, except for brief quotations used in reviews.

SAFETY NOTICE: Although Wilderness Press and the author have made every attempt to ensure that the information in this book is accurate at press time, they are not responsible for any loss, damage, injury, or inconvenience that may occur to anyone while using this book. You are responsible for your own safety and health while engaging in any of the activities described in this book.

Acknowledgments

When I started to write *Camping With Kids*, I set a goal for myself of col-lecting information from at least 100 different individuals. I am grateful to the following 122 people who were kind enough to talk to me or write to me or respond to my emails; to the many anonymous people who shared their experience on the internet; and to the parents who permitted me to photograph their children: Jackie Alexander; Laura Alexander; Amy Anderson, KOA Seattle; Stephanie Arbaugh; Roger Arnell, RV Gold, Oregon; Ranger Jeff Bagshaw, Haleakala National Park, Maui; Raina Ballard; Roberta Bennet; Zach Bennet; Robert A. Boyd; Diana Brement; Clark Carr, Island RV, Kona, Hawaii; Henk and Elke Dawson; Henk Dawson, Jr.; Sarah Essex; Sam Essex; Beth Gendler; Tom Gonser of www.rversonline.org; Ellen Gonser; Bridgit Giedeman; Susan Hankin; Sara Hanneman; Nancy Hanneman; Marlene Haslam; Sandra Lankman Heindsmann; Maggie Herman; Randy Hermans; Sandy Jarvis; Madelaine Jensen; Ava Hamilton Joyrich; Eden Hamilton Joyrich; Andrea Kaawalea, Ethan Katz; Jesse Katz; Volcano National Park Visitors Center, Hawaii; Bill and Jane Kadner; Ruth Kimball; Adam Kimball; Joanne Kloster, *RVLife*; Ricki and Michael Koppel; Kathy Kruger, Washington State Safety Restraint Coalition; Sara, Danielle, and Elana Kupor; Janetta Lee; Holly Levin; Wendy Liebreich, Portland Luggage Co.; Betty Luttrell; Cindy Lynch; Zoe Meyers; Wendy Miller, REI PEAK Program; Jack Mohnhautp, Happy Seat; Chris Morgan, Insight Wildlife Management; Dobbie Norris; Deborah O'Connor; Jennifer Paver, Washington State Safety Restraint Coalition; Joyce Riley; Vicki Robbins; Gloria Roden; Carina Sauerzopf; Barbara Short; Jenny Singer; Robert Singer; Habib Steffen; Kristen Thorstenson, Washington State Safety Restraint Coalition; Christine Underwood; Jeanie Underwood; Nan and Jack Wiseman; Randee Young, the SkiForAll Foundation; 52 sixth and seventh grade students and two teachers at Assumption St. Bridget School in Seattle; and one US Forest Service ranger who didn't want his name used.

I am also deeply indebted to two photographers, Henk Dawson, Jr., and Jon Ostrow, who shared their work with me, and to three mentors, Marcella Benditt, Marion Gartler, and Louise Marshall, who started me writing books. Most of all I am beholden, that old-fashioned word, to my photographer, driver, listener, nurturer, companion, and best friend, my infinitely patient husband, Don.

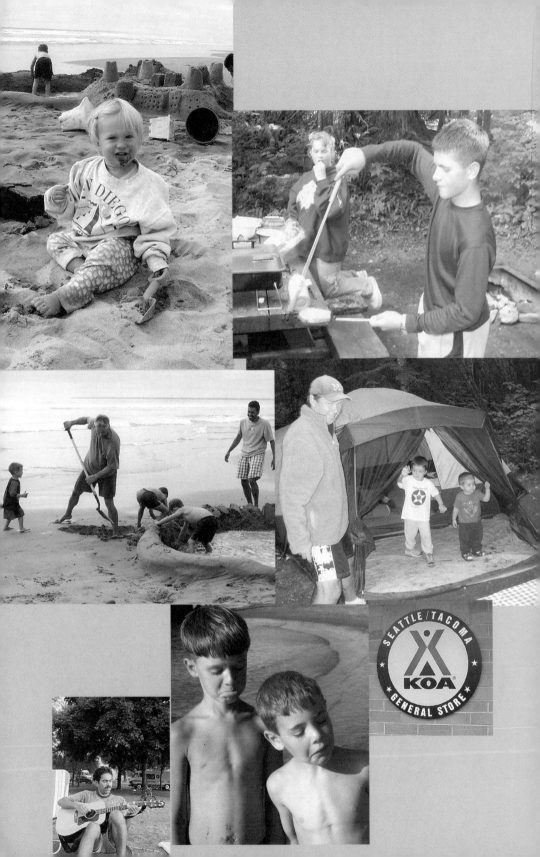

Contents

Preface

I did not grow up in a camping family, but the seeds of an outdoor life must have been planted somehow, because as a young girl I loved no play activity so much as running through the trails at a city park near my home, Elmwood Park in Omaha, Nebraska. My friends and I raced along the dirt paths, back and forth on either side of the creek, crossing at creek level on stepping stones or high in the air on fallen trees or big metal water pipes.

In college, while other couples went off to the movies, the young man who later became my husband and I cooked our dinner in a park or beside a lake on the small, portable grill we always kept in the trunk of his car.

So it should come as no surprise that eventually we should become campers, and when we had children, we camped with them, too.

When my husband was a medical intern and we were new to the Pacific Northwest, his department organized a campout on the Washington coast. We had limited funds. A local store advertised a special on Coleman stoves and lanterns, and since we could afford only one, he asked a coworker which we should buy. The lantern, he was told. Big mistake. We thought we could cook over a fire, but the wood we collected was damp. We never got our fire going beyond smoke. I remember our son Jeff in his red pajamas, sitting in the borrowed tent in a makeshift bed of old comforters over thick layers of newspaper, eating dry Cheerios while we tried to get a breakfast fire started.

A few years later, we were spending all of our family vacations camping with our three children in a rented trailer on the Oregon coast. Our favorite park was Jesse M. Honeyman State Park, a magical place with huge sand dunes almost three stories tall that slope down into clear, ice-cold lakes. We rolled down the dunes, dug in the sand, and hiked across the dunes to the ocean beaches. We told Jeff not to lose his shoes while he was playing in the sand, so he carefully buried them at the side of the dune; we never saw them again.

Sometime along the way, we became backpackers, leaving the car behind. I wrote a book called *Backpacking with Babies and Small Children*. Like this book you are reading, it was based on interviews with many people.

Years later, we went back to Honeyman Park with Jeff, his wife, and our two grandchildren. We set up four tents in two tent sites—each grandkid had to have a tent of his or her own. The grandchildren were much more interested in riding on the dune buggies than in digging or hiking. Daniel, who was 8 at the time, told me he did not like to go places "where you had to walk to get there." Both of the kids preferred going into town for fast food to eating meals cooked outdoors.

Today, all of my children and grandchildren camp. Jeff's family camps in tents next to the car; Judy and John are backpackers. Last summer, our grandson, Daniel, 19 and home from college, accompanied my husband and me on a three-day backpack near Mt. Baker. Daniel carried all the food, the lunches for our dayhikes out of base camp, and he even carried my backpack across the skinny tree that served as a bridge over a wild and rushing stream.

What can you learn from my story? That while it helps to grow up in a camping family, you don't have to camp as a child to be a camper as an adult. That reluctant children can grow up to be enthusiastic campers. That some of the lessons you try to instill in your children don't show up until many years later.

I am a camping grandmother, and I have no intention of quitting. Every Wednesday, I lead an informal group of my friends on a hike somewhere near Seattle. I love nothing so much as a day in the woods or at the beach. I believe that food cooked outdoors always tastes better, and a sleeping bag under the stars is the best of all beds. I am writing this book in order to share with others my love for a simple life spent out of doors, and in the hope that others will learn to share this life with their children, as I have done.

In preparation for writing this book, I talked to a lot of people. I was fortunate to be invited to speak about my work to the sixth- and seventh-grade classes of Assumption St. Bridget School in Seattle. As an assignment following my visit, the students wrote essays about their lifetimes of camping experiences, and they shared their work with me. I also interviewed a number of parents, members of my Jazzercise class, writers from my writing group, and readers from my reading group. I talked to strangers at RV shows and telephoned forest rangers, safety experts, and salespeople at outdoor stores. Altogether, I talked to more than 100 people.

You will notice that throughout the book, I use only first names. I have tried to indicate which comments come from adults and which from students, but in some cases it will not be easy to tell the difference; not surprisingly, children and their parents often shared similar values.

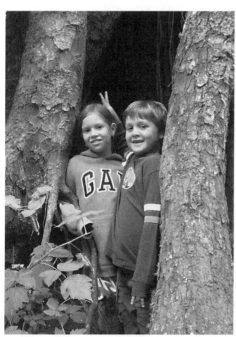

Sarah and Sam, two of my "camping experts," pose for a photo.

I started out thinking of these people as respondents, but as I talked to more and more of them, I realized that they are expert campers; together, they have years and years of camping experience. So when you read, "My experts say..." you will know that you are getting information not just from the printed page, but from someone who has spent time out there under the sun and in the rain and beneath the stars, camping with their families.

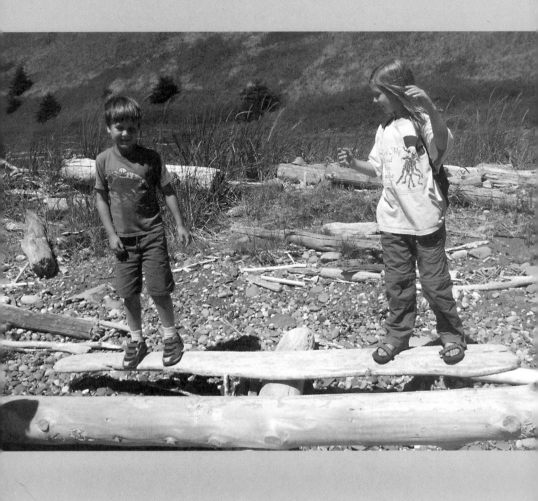

Starting Out

▶ Why Camp?

▶ What's in this Book?

▶ What Kind of Camper Am I?

▶ How Can I Prepare My Family?

Why Camp?

Camping is so much fun! If you have never tried it, you can probably think of all sorts of reasons not to camp, like never having managed a tent or slept on the ground, or your kids are too young, or it's too much work. But balance against all that the wonderful feelings your children will develop about themselves and about their families. Consider some of the good things my student essay writers told me about their camping experiences.

Many of the young people used the word "awesome," this time close to its original meaning, inspiring awe, the feeling of reverence or admiration for that which is grand or sublime or powerful. They also talked of the pleasure of having their parents' undivided attention, and of being outdoors all the time.

Ella, 11, and Stephen, 12, both agreed that when you are camping, you get to spend quality time bonding with your family.

For Shannon, 12, who recalled her first camping trip when she was 8 years old, exploring her camping area with a friend was "as adventurous as two naturalists braving the African jungles alone."

Bridget, 12, wrote that when it was time to leave, "We were all disappointed because camping was so much fun."

Emily and Hannah, both 11, waxed poetic. Emily felt that she was in a "wonderland where you are one with nature." She loved the nights listening to "the chirp of the crickets and grasshoppers and laying down on the ground and looking up at the stars."

Hannah, like Emily, remembered seeing "the stars at night in the crystal-clear sky and never wanting to leave." She also remembered "the smell of everything, the way the air and the pine trees and the way a campfire smelled." And because her family doesn't camp anymore, she has to have "the memories of that one camping trip to last me a lifetime."

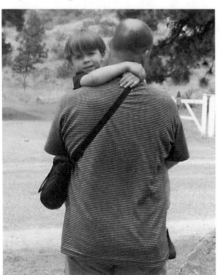

Camping provides quality time with family.

Other students whose families had never taken them camping wished that they could go. "My dad used to camp often with his family when he was young, but no one in our family has been really interested... I think camping would be fun," one young woman wrote, adding that if she could only go camping, she has been thinking about what she would take with her: roller blades or a bike, lots of food, clothes, ingredients for s'mores, and folding chairs, all in an RV.

A young man wrote: "I do not know if I will ever go camping in my life, but I would sure enjoy it."

Contrast those wistful comments with those of Eric, 11: "It was the best time I ever had with my dad."

Why do we take our children camping? For the same reasons we do it ourselves. Camping is a wonderful way for a family to vacation, and it's an opportunity for children and parents to spend time together and get to know each other better. Camping can be luxurious or spare. Camping families may cover many miles or restrict themselves to a single park. The usual rules of hygiene may be followed or relaxed. It can be fun, educational, and economical.

Camping can be a spiritual experience, as it is for Sara and her family, who often read a prayer service together when they are camped on the Sabbath. Or it can be a challenge, as it is for Diana's family, who try to live for a few days with a minimum of material goods. Or it can be an exercise in simplicity, as it is for Madelaine, who says year-round living in a house with all its conveniences is artificial compared to basic living outdoors in a tent. Making a little section of the woods into a home, she says, puts her in touch with ancestors who might have been nomads or cavemen.

Camping is an individual experience. Let's begin your unique adventure.

What's in this Book?

Parents who never camped as children may wish to try it but feel a little reluctant to undertake a new activity that seems so demanding. That's where *Camping with Kids* comes in. I reached out to more than 100 individuals, parents and kids of all ages, to learn how they camped and what they thought about it. Based on their responses, this book will take you, step by step, through the decisions you need to make in order to create your own extraordinary camping experience and cherished family memories.

● ●

How this Book is Organized

▶ Starting Out

▶ Planning Your Trip

▶ The Real Thing

▶ Staying Safe, Sound, and Happy

▶ Beyond Camping: Leaving the Car Behind

● ●

There are five basic sections to *Camping with Kids*. Each section begins with a short list of topics that section will cover. Think of them as my FAQ, frequently asked questions. The first section, Starting Out, is where we are presently. Now that you have decided to try camping, we'll go on to help you decide what kind of camping experience you'll look for and how you will camp, in a tent or a recreation vehicle, also called an RV. Finally, we'll go on to discuss how to help your kids prepare for their adventures in the outdoors, and what to expect of them.

Planning your trip is the topic of the second section. First, we'll find just the right campground for your family's adventure, and we'll tell you how to reserve your place there. Next, we'll go over what you need to take, for your needs in camp and for fun there. This section also covers how to pack for your trip—which can be a challenge when you need to get your entire family and their belongings for the trip into your car. Recognizing that not all of us are the same, a section on special concerns covers topics that range from camping with infants or toddlers to religious observances to camping with a disabled child to taking the dog along.

The third section, The Real Thing, covers your actual camping adventure. We start with the trip to the campground and how to keep the kids happy en route. We'll set up your camp and go over the rules for life in camp. This section includes abundant details on what I learned from other families about good foods for camping. Another extensive section covers fun activities to keep you and the kids busy and entertained, with an emphasis on learning to love the outdoors.

Acknowledging that even the best plans sometimes go awry, the fourth section, Staying Safe, Sound, and Happy, covers what to do when things do not go as planned. One section covers contingency plans and emergencies. Safety on the road and in camp are primary concerns of mine, so I have created separate sections on safety on the road and in camp, dangers, first aid, and what to do if someone is lost.

The last section is Beyond Camping: Leaving the Car Behind. Here we assume that you have developed your car-camping skills in drive-in campgrounds, and you're ready to take your family onto the next stage, backpacking, bike or canoe touring, or other outdoor adventures.

As you read through the sections, you will notice some recurring features. "Expert's Advice" is an especially helpful hint or bit of wisdom from one of the experts who were interviewed for the book. "Helping Hands" indicates an activity in which your children can be involved. When you need to make a decision, a "Quick Quiz" will briefly lay out the alternatives. "Checklist" provides organizing tools to keep you on track. "Imaginary Camping" encourages you to think yourself into a camping situation. Also look for other sidebars throughout the book that highlight important ideas or information.

Look for these Features

 Expert's Advice

 Imaginary Camping

 Helping Hands

 Quick Quiz

 Checklist

What Kind of Camper Am I?

Somewhere near a river, or a lake, or a seashore, in the Northwest, or the Southeast, or New England, at sunset: A light rain is falling. Parents are calling their children in for supper.

At a private campground, three kids are sitting around a table in their motorhome. They have just showered in their self-contained bathroom, and now they're having lasagna, hot from the microwave oven, and a fresh green salad. After they eat, they might wander over to the clubhouse to play Ping-Pong, or they might watch television or a movie.

Down the road, at a public campground, three other kids are crowded around a table in their pop-up tent-trailer. They showered at the bathhouse down the road, and now they are having a thick stew that was prepared at home, carried in a cooler, and warmed on a propane stove. After they eat, they might wander down to the ranger's nightly talk, or they might just stay in their bunks and read by the light of the wall lamps.

Nearby, at the same public campground, three more kids are sitting at a picnic table under a rain fly, eating hot dogs roasted on the fire pit at their campsite. They skipped their shower. After they eat, they, too, might attend the ranger's talk, or they might crawl into the sleeping bags in their tent, where one of their parents will read to them by the light of a headlamp.

If you were to ask any of these children how they spent their vacations, they would all give the same answer: "We were camping."

What is camping? Here's my definition: spending the night up close to nature within a beautiful natural setting. Is staying in a tent in a state or national park camping? Definitely. Is hiking in that same park and going home to sleep camping? No, because you're not staying overnight. Is staying in a hotel or resort within that park or right next to it camping? Not if you have to go down a flight of stairs or cross a lobby to get from your bed to the park. Is sleeping in a yurt, a cabin, or an RV considered camping? If you can step from your temporary home directly out to nature, then yes, you are camping.

So, what kind of camper are you? What can you tolerate? If you need a really comfortable bed to sleep in every night, you should opt for an RV. If you can sleep on an inflated mattress or even on a tarp on the ground, you could camp in a tent. If you must start every day with a hot morning shower and a clean set of clothes, go for the RV. If it doesn't bother you to skip your shower for a day or two or even three, and if you can happily turn your shirt inside out or backward to create a clean shirt front, you can be a tent camper or even a backpacker.

What about meals? Does cooking over an open, smoky fire bring out the caveman or cavewoman in you, the connection to our earliest ancestors, or do you prefer your built-in burners, oven, microwave, and exhaust fan? In the evening, do you eat or dine?

To discover what kind of camper you are, consider the amenities you might find in an RV versus the features of tent camping, and

I M A G I N A R Y   C A M P I N G

What Kind of Camping is Best for You?

To find out what kind of camper you are, practice imaginary camping. As you go through the activities of daily living, brushing your teeth and combing your hair, for example, or getting the kids ready for bed, or preparing meals and then cleaning up afterward, think about how you would carry out those activities in a camp setting. Are you willing to discreetly brush your teeth at a campsite? Could you dress the kids in their pajamas while you were kneeling on the floor of a tent? Imagine yourself carrying out those tasks in the open air with a picnic table and a tent as your only furnishings. Ask yourself: How long would my family be able to live under those circumstances. One night? A week?

Next, try to imagine performing those same tasks, at the same campsite, but with a van or a trailer that provided you with beds and a solid roof overhead. Imagine the same tasks in an RV with a sitting room and a separate bedroom.

Now move your imaginary tent or van or RV from a primitive state park with a lake but no indoor plumbing or hookups, to a plush private campground with a heated swimming pool, a playground, and a recreation center with a game room and movies every night. Ask yourself the same questions: How long would we be able to live under those circumstances. One night? A week?

Which scenario do you see yourself in? Don't answer immediately. Take several days to think about it.

then take an imaginary journey in your mind to decide where you and your family fit best.

RV Amenities

An RV can come with all the appointments of your home kitchen—a refrigerator, freezer, stove, oven, microwave, and exhaust fan. RV campers can dine on gourmet foods, cooked and eaten indoors at a beautifully set table. An RV has built-in couches and a dinette table with benches or chairs. There are lots of cupboards and drawers so you can bring along books and games and other toys. The dinette and some of the couches convert into beds, and there is often another bed in a room of its own, which gives parents a measure of privacy.

RVs usually have kitchen and bathroom sinks, a toilet, a shower (or sometimes a bathtub), and one or more television sets. On long drives, the kids can watch their favorite videos. Some motorhomes have washers and dryers, although many campgrounds do not allow guests to run these appliances because they draw too much current.

Some models of RVs have walls that slide out,

Quick Quiz

What's Your Camp Style?

1. How many clean fronts does a T-shirt have? Circle the right answer: 1 2 3 4

2. A campfire is:
   a. a place to cook dinner.
   b. the center of a social circle.

3. At minimum, a comfortable bed must have:
   a. an inner-spring mattress.
   b. a thin foam pad.
   c. a tarp to cover the bare ground.

4. I can't eat unless I have:
   a. a table set with cloth, napkins, and china dishes.
   b. no flies or mosquitoes.
   c. a chair or bench with a comfortable back.
   d. all of the above.

Answers: If your T-shirt has four clean fronts, if you cook on a campfire, and if you eat and sleep on the ground, you can be a backpacker. If your T-shirt has only one clean front, if you socialize around the fire, if you sleep on a mattress, and if you dine in style, you should choose an RV. Anyone in between can be a tent camper.

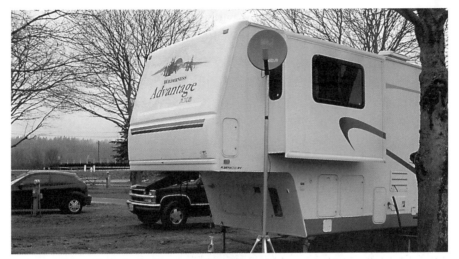

RV amenities might include a satellite dish.

making the interior even larger. On another outside wall, most have an awning, creating a shady haven for lounging or cooking outdoors. Often there is room underneath for bringing along tricycles, bicycles, and scooters.

RVs are self-contained, which means that they carry propane gas for cooking and heating, a water supply for kitchen and bath, batteries for lights and television, and a holding tank for waste from the kitchen and bath. However, most RV campers prefer to park where they have a complete hookup, which means they connect to water, electricity, and sewer. Some private parks have deluxe hookups that also include cable and telephone service, and almost all parks have a dumping station so the holding tank can be emptied.

Features of Tent Camping

Tent campers do not have luxury kitchens. They cook outdoors over a fire or on a one- or two-burner gasoline or propane stove. They bring long-handled tools for roasting hot dogs or marshmallows, and aluminum foil for cooking in the coals. Tent campers store perishable foods in an ice chest and dry foods in a tightly closed container. At night they must store their foods where animals can't get them. Some campgrounds provide creature-proof storage; in others, the food goes back in the car or it's hung from a tree. Tent campers eat at picnic tables, sitting on benches that have no backs. While some bring folding chairs for lounging around the fire, many campers sprawl on the ground.

There are no bathrooms in a tent; you either shower in a bathhouse, if there is one, bathe in a basin, or skip it. Some campgrounds provide flush toilets in the bathhouse, but more primitive camps have only outhouses. Some campers carry portable potties to avoid a long walk to the outhouse in the middle of the night.

Tent campers carry water. Some of them bring big jugs from home. Others walk to a central spigot or pump in camp and carry water back to their campsite. If there is no central water supply, campers will pump and filter water from a lake or a stream and carry it back to camp.

Many campers deliberately choose to live for a few days with the barest minimum of essentials as a way of challenging themselves. In between those campers and those who go for the most luxurious of furnishings, there is a wide variety of opportunities. Campers in trailers, in pop-up tent-trailers with cloth side walls, and in outfitted vans have some of the amenities of the RV campers without the spaciousness. They also have some of the Spartan challenges of the tent campers.

How Can I Prepare My Family?

My friend Vicki has a lovely childhood memory of indoor camping. She had a "campfire" made of crumpled red and yellow tissue paper with a flashlight inside. She remembers eating lunch at her campfire, from a "mess kit" made from a recycled deli container filled with a sandwich, fruit, and snacks. Vicki probably thought this was a game, great fun, but her wise parents were actually preparing her for camping, learning to live in a tent. Preparing your family to camp is actually a learning experience, for you and for them. In this section, we will cover learning to live in a tent and in an RV; we'll go over some ways to learn about nature, with special emphasis on two great programs, PEAK and Leave No Trace; and, finally, we'll learn about campgrounds—they aren't city parks.

Learning to Live in a Tent

A great way to prepare your kids—and yourself—for camping is to practice setting up your tent and letting your kids spend some time inside. You need to practice setting up your tent anyway; later, we'll talk about near disasters that happened to people who tried to make camp when they didn't know how to put the tent up.

If your tent is self-supporting, that is, if it doesn't need to be pegged down, you can set it up in the family room or play room. Let your young children nap inside the tent. If your tent is set up out-

IMAGINARY CAMPING

Camping at Home

Help your kids "experience" camping before you go by practicing camping at home. Make a tent by spreading a blanket over a low table or a chair tipped on its side. Let them spend time inside this smaller space, which will have the same feel as a tent.

side, don't just put it up and take it down, but leave it up for a while. Eat a meal outside next to or inside the tent. Perhaps you can even spend a night, or part of a night, sleeping outside.

Talking about the tent in advance and putting it up at home before your trip could avert a problem when night falls in camp. Many campers can tell you horror stories of being kept awake by a crying child two or even three campsites away from theirs. I can't emphasize this enough: Practicing with the tent is a wise idea on two counts—you need to know how to do it, and young children need to feel that it's a familiar space.

If you don't have access to a tent, improvise. When my brothers and I were little, one of our favorite games was "covered wagon." Every Saturday, we tipped our big rocking chair over and spread a blanket over the rockers. The room inside the blanket could just as easily been called a tent. If you don't have a rocking chair, make

your tent from a blanket and a card table or a low table or a
tipped-over chair. Let your kids take a nap in their tent or take
their favorite stuffed animals inside and tuck them in for a "nap."

Learning to Live in an RV

If you're planning to camp in an RV, you can also spend some
days and even nights in it, if it's parked at home. If you haven't yet
acquired the RV, whether you plan to rent or buy (more on this
later), you can stop at an RV sales lot with your kids and walk
through a few models.

If you're driving somewhere where your route takes you past an
RV sales lot, plan to leave an hour early to allow time to check out
the RVs. Walk through the different models and show the kids
where the bed is over the cab, if it's that kind of arrangement, how
the dinette folds down to make another bed, where the range and
refrigerator are, where the toilet and the shower are located. Talk
about who might sleep in each bed, and how you will eat breakfast
after the dinette is folded into place again.

Don't be shy about visiting RV lots more than once. Sales people
in RV lots should welcome you as potential future customers.

Learning About Nature

At the same time you and your children are preparing to eat your
meals and spend the night out of doors, you can be getting ready
for the up-close-to-nature adventure of camping. Remember my definition of camping: spending the night up close to nature within a
beautiful natural setting. Your goal is to make your children comfortable and curious in the out of doors.

You can begin to study nature in your own neighborhood. Start
by taking "hikes" in your local park. Carry a magnifying glass for
an up-close look at plants and insects. Older children can record
their findings in a small notebook or tablet, or draw pictures with
colored pencils. If you have a digital camera, let them use it to
record what they see for their very own nature CD.

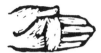

H E L P I N G   H A N D S

Mini Museum

Your children will gain interest in nature and the things you might see on your camping trip if you help them start a "museum." Encourage your children to pick up interesting specimens on your hikes and clear a shelf or table top to display these interesting finds at your home.

Take time to look at the plants that grow around you. Examine the way plants change in the course of just a few weeks, from bud to flower to seed. Find the stump of a tree that was cut and count the rings. How old was that tree when it was cut? Measure the tree's circumference and diameter. (These are good words to teach your 9- and 10-year-old children, but for 6- or 7-year-olds, just explain how many inches the tree is across or around.) You'll need to carry a tape measure.

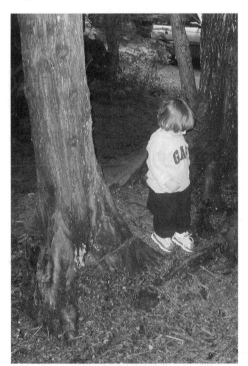

A simple walk to find cones and pretty leaves teaches kids about nature.

A visit to a pond or a lake can be an opportunity to look at rocks on the shore: How many different colored rocks can you find? Bundle up on a rainy day and go out to look for animal tracks—dogs, cats, squirrels, birds—in the mud. Or make your own tracks and study them. Who has the biggest track? Who has the most distinguished tracks? Why are some tracks deeper than others?

The birds and "wild animals" in your neighborhood are another focus for nature study. How many different kinds of birds can you see?

How many squirrels? Can you catch a butterfly or a flying bug in a net? Look at the butterflies you see and draw pictures of them. Look at the way butterflies and other flying bugs move through the air. Remember the boxer who "danced like a butterfly?" Can you and your children dance like a butterfly?

Where you live, do you have the ducks, Canada geese, raccoons, and possums that I have in my urban Seattle neighborhood? If not, a trip to the zoo may be in order, not to look at exotic animals but to concentrate on the locals.

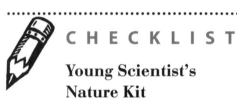

CHECKLIST

Young Scientist's Nature Kit

▶ Magnifying glass

▶ Notebook and pencils

▶ Colored pencils

▶ Camera

▶ Tape measure

▶ Butterfly net

▶ Flashlight

▶ Binoculars

These in-city excursions are good times to begin teaching your children respect for nature. They can look at the animals, but they should not chase them, feed them, or pick them up. They should learn to look at but not pick the plants. On the other hand, if something is already detached and lying on the ground, such as a pine cone or a pretty rock, it is permissible to pick it up.

Let your child start a "museum" at home of interesting specimens he or she has collected on your walks. Set aside a shelf or a table top for the collection. Be sure to return those items to the park when you clear the shelf

Since your camping trip will include nights spent out of doors, take some of your nature hikes at night. Look at the full moon with binoculars. Look at the stars. A 5-year-old might be able to learn to recognize the Big and Little Dippers. With help, older children could find other constellations. Older children can also track the phases of the moon, from new to full and back to new again.

Step into the backyard at night or go to a safe park and listen. What can you hear? At my house, I hear ducks quacking and geese honking as they fly by. Keep a night journal of what you see and hear. Use a flashlight to look at, and under, the plants in your yard. Are there insects there that you didn't see during the day? Can you find a moth? Moths are creatures of the night, while butterflies are seen during the day. Moths spread their wings out flat, while resting butterflies generally hold their wings up straight.

Sometimes the out of doors can be studied indoors. Parents who are feeling intimidated at the idea of all this nature study because they have no background for it can accompany their kids to the closest library. Spend an afternoon browsing through the books on birds, bugs, rocks, flowers, and plants. Younger children will be content to look at the pictures. Older children can select some books to take home. Ask the librarian for help finding the books appropriate for the age and interest of your children. While you're there, look at the books on camping, too.

Is there a museum of science or natural history near your home? Is there a botanical garden or a greenhouse in a public park? An ecology center? An outdoor store? Any of those places will have displays or exhibits that you can use to say, "This is what we might see when we're camping."

> ## Quick Quiz
>
> ### Nature Study
>
> **Q:** How many places are there near your home where you can begin to study nature?
>
> **A:** Your yard, the library, the park, the science museum, a botanical garden.

PEAK and Leave No Trace

REI, the outdoor retail cooperative, and Leave No Trace (LNT), an organization that teaches responsible outdoor recreation, have joined together to offer a program they call Promoting Environmental Awareness in Kids, or PEAK. PEAK is based on the seven principles of Leave No Trace (see page 17).

REI will send staff members or volunteers to speak to your child's class or youth group or even birthday party. A PEAK presentation is made up of several different activities. Wendy Miller, events and outreach coordinator at the REI in Seattle, told me about an activity called the Web of Life that has been very popular in our area. This activity introduces the seven principles through a game in which kids use cards around their necks to trace the food chain, from mosquito to salmon to bear. For other presentations, the REI representative may bring a backpack containing camping equipment useful for responsible camping, like a trowel for digging a hole for your human waste, or a bear bag for storing food out of the reach of animals.

Contact the REI store nearest you (find one by calling 800-426-4840 or visiting www.rei.com) to arrange an age-appropriate presentation for your group. Visits can last one to two hours. You can learn more about Leave No Trace on their website, www.lnt.org, or by calling 800-332-4100. I believe that every family should adopt these principles as their personal outdoor creed. You will find these ideas repeated many times through this book.

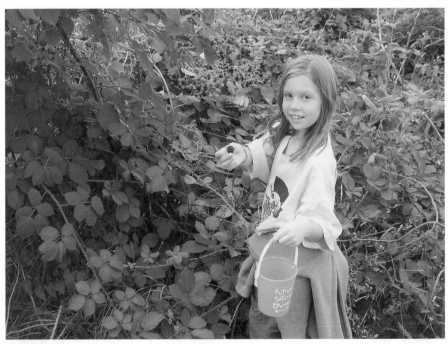

Following the principles of Leave No Trace means leaving what you find, but picking the occasional blackberry is OK.

Principles of Leave No Trace

1. **Know before you go:** Be prepared with the right clothes and equipment. Know how you are going to camp and something about the area. Read Planning Your Trip, page 23.

2. **Choose the right path:** Stay on the trail. Do not walk on wildflower meadows or areas that have been marked for rehabilitation. Choose a campground that has the features you want, and, once you're there, camp in a designated campsite. Read the sections Where Shall We Go?, page 41, and What if Someone is Lost?, page 216.

3. **Trash your trash:** Put all litter in trash cans or carry it home. Carrying it home is better than leaving it in camp; some park budgets have been cut so drastically that trash is not picked up as often as it should be. If there is no bathroom or outhouse, bury your poop in a hole 4 to 8 inches deep and 100 big steps from any stream or lake. (Leave No Trace assumes that a "big step" is 2 feet long, for a total of 200 feet away from water.) Carry your toilet paper out in a plastic bag. Keep water clean. Do not put soap, food, or any other waste in lakes or streams. Read the section What's Life in Camp Really Like?, page 139.

4. **Leave what you find:** Here, I disagree a little bit with LNT guidelines. I think it's OK to collect rocks on the beach and leaves or plant material that have already fallen, unless they are special plants, like cones from sequoia trees. Treat living plants with respect. Leave historical items as you found them so the next person can enjoy them. Don't dig trenches or build structures in your campsite. Read the section What Should We Do for Fun?, page 170.

5. **Be careful with fire:** Before you build a campfire, check fire regulations and restrictions for the local area. Use a fire ring that's already in place and keep your fire small. Do not take branches from living trees; collect only loose sticks on the ground. Be sure the fire is completely cold and out before you leave. Read the section called How Do We Cook in Camp?, beginning on page 153.

6. **Respect wildlife:** Observe animals from a distance and never approach, chase, or feed them. Human food is unhealthy for animals; feeding them will start them on bad habits. Store your food and trash so animals can't get to them. Control pets at all times or leave them at home. Reread the paragraphs on animals in this section, and read the paragraphs in the relevant sections in What's Life in Camp Really Like? (page 139), How Do We Cook in Camp? (page 153), and What Should We Do for Fun? (page 170).

7. **Be kind to other visitors:** Make sure the fun you have does not bother anyone else. Remember that other campers may be there to enjoy the peace and quiet of the outdoors. Avoid making loud noises or yelling. See the section on good manners in camp on page 148.

Learning about Campgrounds

When John Silverman was in pre-school, he was part of a group of children who were chosen to appear on a local children's television program. He had watched this program many times. We took him to the studio, he looked around, and he said, "This isn't what I thought it would be. Where is the little box?"

You and your children may have had a lot of conversations about camping, but the kids' perceptions of what a campground is like may be a little bit skewed. It's not your backyard! Try to find a park

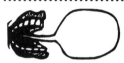

E X P E R T ' S   A D V I C E

Fun for Everyone

Everyone should have the opportunity to say what she or he would like to do while camping. When you're finally in camp, make sure that you actually do at least one of the things that each person asked for. Hugh, who is 12, told me, "Before we went on the trip, it was important that my dad researched the area to see if it would be fun not only for us but for him, too."

near your home that allows camping, and walk through it. Point out the fire pits, the picnic tables, and the platforms for tents or RVs. Show them the bathrooms or outhouses. If you're going to be camping at a private campground, visit the KOA campground closest to your home. Look at their bathrooms, playgrounds, and pool, if there is one.

When you begin to plan the logistics of your camping trips, include the kids. Let them look at the maps of the states you will be visiting. Siblings can work together on this project. Even young pre-readers can find the little green trees or the red tents on the map that designate parks with camping. Older children can make lists of the parks they find.

When you send away for information about camping opportunities, ask to have the information sent to your kids' names. They can have the thrill of a big packet of mail arriving just for them. If you have asked for material for children, they may find Junior Ranger or Smokey Bear pamphlets included. Young children can look at the pictures and all of you can talk about all the fun things you will do together. Make sure that everyone has the opportunity to say what she or he would like to do while camping.

Websites for Kids

Older kids can begin to research your camping trip on the web. If they go to www.50states.com, they can learn a lot about the state they will be visiting. If they go to the National Park Service site, www.nps.gov, they can learn about the national park, monument, seashore, historic site, or forest that you will be visiting.

They can also become Junior Rangers or WebRangers. Official Junior Rangers are programs in state and national parks, but your kids can learn about them before you leave home. Just go to www.nps.gov/learn/juniorranger.htm, or ask your browser for Junior Ranger. Or, if you go to the National Park Service's website, www.nps.gov, first click on Interpretation and Education, and then click on GoZONE.

C H E C K L I S T

Websites for Kids

▶ Information about states: www.50states.com
▶ Information about national parks: www.nps.gov
▶ Information about Junior Rangers: www.nps.gov/learn/juniorranger.htm
▶ Information about WebRangers: www.nps.gov/webrangers

If you don't have access to a computer, use your local library to research the states and the parks you will visit. Have your children call the office of the national park that interests you. The ranger I spoke to at Mt. Rainier National Park assured me that they would mail the Junior Ranger booklet or other educational packets to anyone who called. For programs in state parks, call or go to the park information center for that state, just as you will do when you are seeking information about camping in that state.

While the Junior Ranger program is for visitors to the parks, WebRanger is a National Park Service program for stay-at-homes. It begins and ends at your computer desk. By logging onto www.nps.gov/webrangers, your child can explore the national parks, complete activities, and win awards. Programs are age appropriate, 6 to 9, 10 to 12, and 13 and up, and new activities are added often. The kids will be learning about natural science and American history while they are having fun. It's a good way to get them excited about and prepared for upcoming trips, or even to help plan next year's trip. WebRanger allows kids to learn about national parks even if they can't visit them, and they send a strong message about caring for our parks and our world.

Some parks have their own websites, with pictures of the facilities, including campsites. This is another place for imaginary camping. Look at the pictures with your kids and talk about how you might camp there.

Finally, when you talk to your kids about camping, make sure that your questions don't mislead them. If you ask what they would like

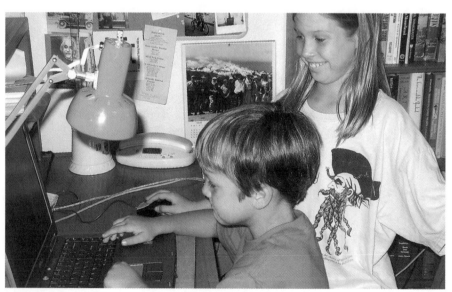

Sam and Sarah like to research their camping trips online.

to eat when camping, they may request something that would be very difficult or impossible to prepare on a camp stove. If you ask which toys they will take, they may list something like Lego, which has a lot of small pieces that would be scattered all over a campsite.

IMAGINARY CAMPING
Campsite Specifics

Look at the various camping websites and find some with photos of campgrounds. After reviewing those, talk with your children about how they would imagine camping at these places. Ask them what they would eat while camping, and what toys they would bring. Of the activities described on the website, what would they do during the day?

Instead, be very specific. When you're having mac and cheese, you can ask, "Would you like to have this when we're camping?" When you're picking up or putting away toys, you can say, "Teddy can go camping with us, but maybe Barbie should stay home (unless there is a Camping Barbie)."

You may be surprised to see your small children begin to incorporate what you have told them into their play. Babies will be babies no matter what you tell them, but toddlers and pre-schoolers might begin to tell their dolls and stuffed animals that they are going camping. Teddy bears can "camp" under a tent made from a favorite blanket.

When I was asked to write this book, my grown daughter gave me a toy camping set made by Danny First. It has a little tent, two cloth dolls (boy and girl), two air mattresses, two sleeping bags, an inflatable boat, and a collection of animals—a skunk, a moose, and a raccoon. Children who have visited me, as young as 2, even the kids who have never camped, seem to understand immediately how to play with the set. A clever parent could replicate some of the items with toys your children already own and a sleeping bag made of a washcloth or a square of felt folded in half and stitched together on two sides.

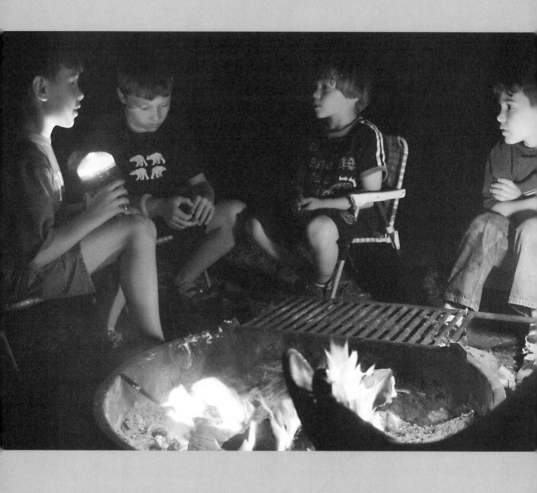

Planning Your Trip

▶ How Shall We Camp?

▶ Where Shall We Go?

▶ What Do We Need?

▶ What About Our
Special Concerns?

How Shall We Camp?

Eleven-year-old Sara camps with her father and younger sister in a four-person tent; sometimes, but not often, their mother goes with them. Susan, her husband, and their four kids camp in two small tents, a parents' tent and a kids' tent. Ever since her daughter was only 3 years old, single parent Janetta has been taking her camping, sometimes just the two of them, in a tent that sleeps five; it's roomy enough to hold the play pen that was her daughter's bed when she was small. Marlene, another single mom, and her two kids, 7 and 9, sleep in the back of their big SUV, with down pillows and comforters; they use their tent only for storage and for changing clothes.

Jeannie and Porter also began camping with their daughter when she was just a toddler, but they camped in a pop-up tent-trailer, which has a floor and a hard lid that pops up to form the roof over canvas walls. Henk Jr. and his wife and kids, 1 and 3, also camp in a pop-up tent-trailer, but when the kids go with their grandparents, Henk Sr. and Elke, they camp in an RV.

Ellen and her family are co-owners with her sister-in-law of a cab-over RV, a truck with living quarters that extend over the driver's cab. They alternate camping weekends with the other family, and once every summer they negotiate for a longer trip. Ellen's RV is "pretty much complete." They leave it packed and ready to go all the time.

Meeghan, a 12-year-old student, hasn't tried it yet, but she thinks an RV would be the best way to camp, because it would be more comfortable and easier to cook in than a tent and she wouldn't have to go home if it rained.

So how will *you* camp? This chapter will help you decide, with detailed discussions of tents, RV camping, trailers, camper trucks, and vans. We'll also cover renting, and, since I know I can't answer all the questions you might have, a short segment on some good sources of further information.

Tents

My family camped in tents most of the time, especially on weekend jaunts. We liked tents because we could pretend that we were rugged outdoor people, getting close to nature, challenging ourselves to live without civilized amenities for just a few days. We slept in sleeping bags on thin mattresses and cooked outdoors on a gasoline stove. We carried water from a spigot in the campground, if there was one, or we pumped water through a filter from a lake or stream.

Although we tried to get along with a minimum of equipment, we often had too much gear for the trunk and the top of the car, so some of it rode with the kids in the back seat. That's not unusual for tent campers. It made for cramped seating, and we tried to stop occasionally to let the kids get out in a safe place and run around. We learned early on that it's important to load the car so that the tent can be taken out first and set up before we did anything else.

We now own several tents. The largest sleeps four close together, with no room for storage inside; when we use this tent, we leave our stove out on the picnic table all night, but most of our gear and our food stays locked in the car. I like this tent because I can stand up in it, and it has a little extension in the front where the dog can sleep. When the whole family camped, one of the kids spent the night by himself in a pup tent. Both tents must be pegged down in order to stay up.

Our second tent is self-supporting, which means that we can set it up in an open area and then carry it to the place where we want it. Sometimes we are surrounded by brush, with only the door opening

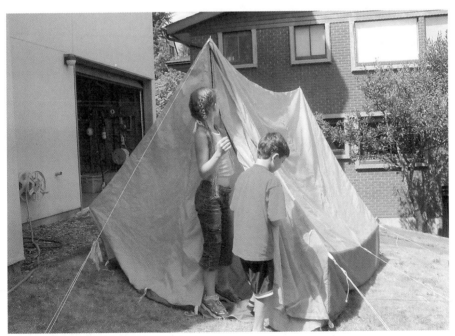

Practice, practice, practice setting up your tent!

to a clear area. We can sleep two or three in this tent, but again, there is no room for storage. This tent stands alone, but once it's in place we peg it down so the wind doesn't blow it away.

Our smallest tent, a backpacker's tent, sleeps only two, but we have to take turns sitting up. It's hard to crawl into this tent and really difficult to change clothes inside. It has to be pegged down to be set up. It is a very lightweight tent, which is important when you're backpacking.

All of our tents have rain flies, and we have added a clothesline inside from one point to the other, where we hang the clothes we take off at night. We also have a pocket sewn into one of the side seams, where we stash our glasses at night.

Most tents are much larger than ours. Some of the largest have side rooms opening off the main room. Michael refers to his tent as a "condo." It has three rooms, with curtains separating them. A tent with a peaked roof provides headroom so you can stand up and walk around inside. Dome-shaped tents come in all sizes. The largest have ample floor space, but you can stand up only in the center. Still, there is room enough inside for low camp cots if you don't like sleeping on the ground, and there's plenty of storage. Many dome-shaped tents are self-supporting. Some manufacturers advertise a "bathtub floor." This means that the waterproofing on the floor of the tent extends up the sides several inches, keeping the tent floor drier in case of rain.

In the Northwest, where I live, most tents come with a rain fly, which is a cover over the tent with an air space between it and the tent roof. Rain and dew collect on the outside of the fly, and moisture exhaled by the people sleeping in the tent collects on the

C H E C K L I S T

Questions to Ask When Choosing a Tent

▶ Is it big enough for my family?
▶ Is it easy to put up?
▶ Is it self-supporting? Does that matter to me?
▶ Can I stand up inside?
▶ How much gear can I store inside?
▶ Does it have a rain fly?

inside of the fly and not on the tent. Some campers carry extra tarps to use as dining flies, to protect their picnic table and cooking area from the dew and the rain. They tie the tarp to trees or to their tent or even to the car, if there's no other place to tie it. If you're camping in a dry, sunny area, you might want the extra fly to provide shade.

You will also see tents advertised as "three-season" or "four-season." There is no national standard for designating seasonality to a tent, but in general, four-season tents have better protection against the elements, heavier coating on the floors, extra reinforcement around zippers and stress points, rain flies that extend farther beyond the tent, and better ventilation (to keep moisture from condensing inside). They are also more expensive. A family camping in the late spring, summer, or early autumn should not need a four-season tent.

If I were starting to tent camp all over again with my family, I'd

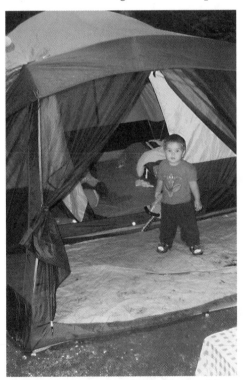

buy a tent like the one I saw last summer when I was walking around a Forest Service campground talking to families with children. It had two rooms, an inner one and outer one. The outer room was screened on three sides. It had a zippered door to the outside, and another zippered door to the inner room. The outer room functioned as a mud room; it had a fabric floor where the two little boys were playing amid a stack of shoes. The inner room, the sleeping room, was kept relatively clean because all the

Tents with two rooms keep dirt outside. shoes were left outside.

We buy all of our tents on sale at the beginning of the season (last year's model) or at an end-of-season clearance. Prices for tents vary considerably. A family tent, which can accommodate six to eight people, advertised in my latest REI sale catalog, is $260, reduced from $350. Campmor, a discount outfit that issues a popular catalogue, lists family tents for four or more at $100, $120, $150, or $190. Larger tents from Campmor that sleep six to eight are $260 and $330. Your local outdoor store or warehouse outlet will often have deals as good as or better than these.

If you're a garage sale or thrift shop fan, you can often find good deals on a used tent. Some communities hold gear swaps, another good source for a used tent, but remember it's buyer beware when you buy a used tent.

Sometimes a friend is willing to lend a tent, so you can try camping before you spend any money. Some people are reluctant to share their outdoor equipment because it requires good care.

In that case, you may have to rent. (See the section on renting on page 38.) Rental fees for tents will vary with the size of the tent and the season; expect to pay more if you rent over a holiday weekend. My most recent REI price list gave the fee of $28 for the first day

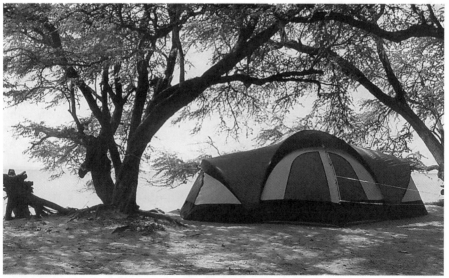

A spacious three-room tent sleeps six to eight.

and $14 for each additional day for a five- to six-person tent. Prices may have gone up since then. In addition to REI, many of your local sporting goods and outdoor stores will rent tents and camping equipment. Wherever you rent, don't expect a lot of choices; you have to be content with what's available. If you rent for your first trip and plan to continue camping, it might be wise to put your rental fees toward your purchase.

Regardless of the size of the tent you plan to take, or whether it's rented, bought, or borrowed, you should practice setting it up outside on your lawn or in a park before you go. In fact, it's a good idea to put it up and take it down several times, so that you won't get into a situation like Maggie did on her first trip. Her family arrived at the campground late, and they had to set up an unfamiliar tent in the dark, trying to read the instructions by flashlight.

Tents are fine in the summer, but if you're planning a camping trip in the fall or early spring, you and especially your children might find the tent inadequate. You may need a more substantial home away from home, like a motorhome or a camper with a heater or at least some protection from the wind.

Some years ago, my husband and our youngest son went off to the mountains in early autumn for a father-son weekend with Indian Guides, a program of the YMCA. They were guests in a camper truck. During the night, the temperature dropped below freezing, and the groceries in the truck—bananas, oranges, bread, sitting outside on the counter—froze solid, but the milk, inside the well-insulated cooler, remained liquid.

On another, longer vacation some years ago, my family rented a travel trailer that we hitched to a station wagon. When we stopped for a few days, we unhitched the trailer and left it in camp while we went off exploring in the wagon. We found the trailer cozy during the rainy nights on the Oregon coast, but when we cooked inside on the propane stove, all the windows ran with moisture.

That was a long time ago. Today, there are many more options for shelter, depending on what you require for comfort and what you can afford to pay.

RV Camping

An RV can be one of several kinds of rolling homes. The critical component is that all have wheels. RVs are self-contained, which means that they carry propane gas for cooking and heating, a water supply for kitchen and bath, batteries for lights, microwave and exhaust fan, and a holding tank for waste from the kitchen and bath. Some have a "dual fuel" refrigerator, which runs on electricity or propane. Others have slide-out walls that zoom out to create more living space when they are parked.

C H E C K L I S T

Questions to Ask About RVs

▶ Is it large enough for my family?

▶ Where will everyone sleep?

▶ Where will everyone ride?

▶ Who will drive it or how will it be towed?

▶ Does it have all the features that I want—kitchen, bath, connections?

▶ Does it have too many conveniences, way beyond roughing it?

The most luxurious of RVs is the motorhome, a small or sometimes not so small, bus or van where the driver's compartment is open to the living space. But an RV can also be a trailer or a living unit—a camper mounted on a pick-up truck.

In a motorhome, passengers ride in the living areas. Sometimes there is a second set of swivel chairs, with seat belts, behind the driver and co-pilot. There is more leg room and "wiggle room" in these spaces than there is in a conventional automobile, and children who tend to poke each other in the car can be separated more easily. Motorhomes have one or more television sets, which some parents find useful in keeping the kids occupied during long drives.

When you stop for the night with a motorhome, you don't just park it. You have to level it, with jacks or ramps, so that all the appliances will work properly. On some models, the jacks are part of the frame. It's easier to do this leveling if your campsite has a concrete pad, but in more primitive campgrounds you may have to park on dirt or gravel.

When the RV campers stop, they prefer the kind of park where they have a complete hook-up, which means they connect to water, electricity, and sewer, although some sites have only water and electricity. Some private parks also provide phone, internet, and cable TV connections. If the RV campers must take a campsite without a sewer or water hook-up, they can use the park's water and bathroom facilities. Some campers pull out portable generators that run on gasoline to power their motorhomes when there is no electrical connection. Other campers sometimes complain that these generators are too noisy, but I was assured by the dealers at the RV show that the new models are quiet. Still, most parks have hours when the generators can't be run.

Because they are self-contained, RV campers are also able to stop in areas with no facilities at all. They call this kind of camping "dry camping," which means that they are totally dependent on the gas, water, and batteries that they carry to supply all their needs. I once

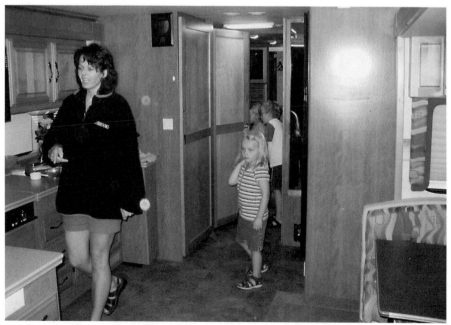

Many motorhomes have luxurious interiors.

saw an RV, obviously occupied, parked on a street in San Francisco early in the morning, but most dry campers are like my friend Deborah. Deborah and her family are hikers. They like to park their RV at the end of the road where several trails lead off into the mountains. Every day, they hike up to a different destination, and then come down again to spend the night in their RV.

Dry campers must calculate very carefully how they use their resources. One long shower could empty the water tank. Too long a stay without a stop at a dumping station might overload their waste-holding tank. Deborah carries a water filter so they can augment their water supply by pumping water from a lake or stream for cooking and drinking, and showers are strictly limited.

When you stop for the night with a motorhome, your vehicle stops with you. You can't take off to go exploring unless you are towing a second vehicle. Our friend Henk refers to the small sedan he pulls as his "dinghy," likening it to the little boat attached to a big cruiser. On steep mountain grades when the motorhome is working hard, they detach the dinghy and his wife drives it until they reach more level ground. Like most drivers who tow a small car, Henk prefers to camp at a site that is a pull through, meaning that he can drive straight ahead when he leaves. It's hard to back up a big motorhome, and even harder with the dinghy attached. Henk warned that not all cars can be used as dinghies. Some with automatic transmissions can't be towed and need to be carried on a trailer; check the owner's manual of your vehicle for instructions on how it should be towed.

Renting an RV is not inexpensive. One national company I consulted had summer rates beginning at $157 per day for the smallest motorhome that sleeps four, with a minimum rental of seven days. Rates went down to $140 per day for the same vehicle for 11 days or longer. Another company advertised longer motorhomes that have slide-outs and sleep seven for $225 per night, with a three-night minimum. These fees did not include mileage charges beyond the daily maximum, personal furnishings, taxes, or campground fees, which range from free in some undeveloped forest areas to $25 and up in private campgrounds. (See more about renting at the end of this section, page 38.)

In addition, there is the cost of fuel; depending on size, RVs get 8 to 12 miles per gallon of fuel. To buy that smallest motorhome that sleeps four, used, with 90,000 miles, but inspected, refurbished, and backed with a limited warranty, the company asks $24,995, or $257 per month. A new one would be even more.

Remember that the RV you buy must be stored someplace when you're not using it, and that may be an additional cost. A storage lot in Seattle charges by the foot for a locked, outside yard. Their minimum for a 20-foot vehicle is $95 per month. After that, they add $4.50 per foot per month.

Trailers

Leaving your "home" to go exploring isn't a problem with a trailer. You can unhitch the towing vehicle and drive into town, leaving your home behind. Vacation homes that are towed are either travel trailers or fifth wheels. A trailer is hitched to the frame of a vehicle, either a truck, SUV, or sedan, but the fifth wheel can only be attached to the bed of a pick-up truck.

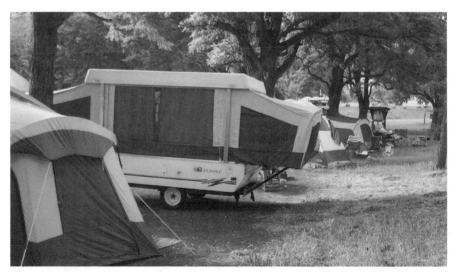

A tent-trailer combines the best features of a tent and trailer.

Large models of these towed homes are very similar to the motorhome, with plumbing and electrical systems, awnings, kitchens, microwaves, and TV sets, and they also need to be leveled when they are parked in camp. A difference is that motorhomes open directly into the driver's compartment; if you have a trailer, you have to leave the driver's compartment and walk outside in order to enter the living space.

Designers of these trailers, like those who design motorhomes, create different floor plans to accommodate varying lifestyles. There is often an extension over the towing vehicle where two people can sleep, with a small ladder leading up to it. Kids tell me they really like to sleep on the raised bunk. Other furnishings inside the trailer fold up or out of the way to provide more beds. According to Matthew, who is 11, "Trailer camping is the ultimate way to spend the summer."

The heavier your trailer is, the beefier your towing vehicle must be. If you're renting a trailer, the agent will want to know how you plan to tow it, and he may reject your car if it isn't powerful enough. SUVs, vans and sedans can pull some, but not all trailers, but as the trailers become smaller, the amenities are fewer. The smallest of trailers will have only enough space for sleeping and

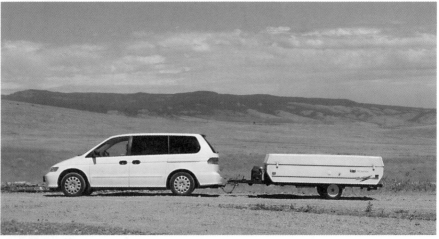

Ordinary passenger cars can tow lightweight tent-trailers.

storage, and possibly a cooler and a chemical toilet, but even a compact car can pull them.

Like motorhomes, the price of a trailer will vary considerably, depending on its size and the amenities inside. In a recent issue of *RVLife*, I saw used trailers advertised as starting at $9500, but some went above $32,000, and many advertisers did not list price at all. The rental for a trailer from one national company was $89 per night for a trailer that sleeps five, to $109 per night for one that sleeps up to eight. Taxes, propane refueling, and a rented trailer hitch are additional costs.

A pop-up or tent-trailer is a kind of hybrid. It's a neat, low, solid-looking unit when it is being towed. Once it's parked in camp, the solid top goes up, fabric walls with sewn-in screens rise, and two or three of the sides pop out to create beds. Although it seems like a tent, it's a whole lot easier to set up, and the smooth and level floor is bare of little rocks and twigs poking through. There's lots of room to store things on the floor of the pop-up, even when the top is down and secure. Some models have additional storage compartments accessible from the outside of the unit. Pop-ups come with kitchens; some even have chemical toilets and collapsible shower stalls. These units are much lighter than other trailers, so ordinary passenger cars can tow them.

Pop-ups need to be leveled too, and, even then, walking in the trailer feels like rolling in a boat. Sleeping in a pop-up trailer is almost like sleeping in a tent, except that you have a big, comfortable bed instead of a skinny cot or hard ground. When my friend Christine was an infant, her mother told me, they put her in one of the big beds and piled clothing and duffels on the edge to keep her from rolling out.

Like the people in big motorhomes, trailer campers prefer pull-through campsites. Backing a trailer into its space is really tricky. Gloria told me that her husband never did get the hang of backing up their pop-up tent-trailer. She did it easily, she said, and their 9-year-old son was expert at leveling it.

If you'd like to rent a tent trailer, you'll have to do a lot of research on the internet and in your local directories. Not many rental agencies carry them. If you choose to buy a tent-trailer, you'll find it more expensive than a tent, but less than a trailer. At a recent RV show that I attended, the most minimal tent-trailer, one that could be towed by a passenger car, sold for only $1500. A salesman who assured me that his tent trailers were "top of the line" told me their prices ranged from $6000 to $16,000. Before you buy one, be sure you have space to store it.

Truck Campers

A truck camper is like a trailer set on the chassis of a pick-up truck. It, too, may have a sleeping area over the cab. These units are popular with rental agencies. Zach liked the fact that his bed was always available, without having to be converted from a sofa or a dinette. Campers tend to be quite compact, but the manufacturers manage to include kitchens, bathrooms, and ingenious storage and sleeping arrangements. On some units, the whole back wall opens up and a ramp slides out, creating a "garage" where you can tie down a motorcycle, an all-terrain vehicle, or a powered wheelchair.

You often see truck campers towing boats or trailers full of motorcycles or bicycles, but like the motorhome, if you want to drive a camper into town, you're taking your home with you. Unlike motorhome drivers, whose compartment is open to the living quarters, camper drivers must leave their seats and walk around the back to enter.

An additional concern with a camper is space for the travelers. Unless the cab of the camper has a back seat, there is no space for the family. Ellen's children like to ride in the bed over the cab of their camper, which she allows on country roads, but on freeways they sit in the back seat of the big cab.

When they were smaller, Ellen's children shared a bed in the camper or slept outside in a tent with a parent. Now her 10-year-old sleeps leaning back in the front seat of the cab while her 9-year-old sleeps in the bed made up from the dinette, and the parents get the over-the-cab bed.

There is a toilet in their camper, but Ellen limits its use. "There's only so much you want to deal with," she explained. If the camp they are visiting has hook-ups and a dumping station, they dump on arrival before attaching the sewage hose. If there is no hook-up, they encourage the use of the camp toilet facilities, and dump just before they leave.

Even though their camper is smaller as RVs go, each member of the family has a cupboard for his or her own clothing, and there's a big bag for dirty clothes. There's also ample room for fishing gear, the scooter, books, and horseshoes.

If you already have a pick-up truck, you can add a fully equipped new camper to it for only $8000, an ad in *RVLife* assures me. This does not include installation. Otherwise, add the cost of the truck of your choice to the price of the camper.

Vans

Another kind of RV that you see less often in the RV shows and in camps is the van that has been converted to or outfitted as a

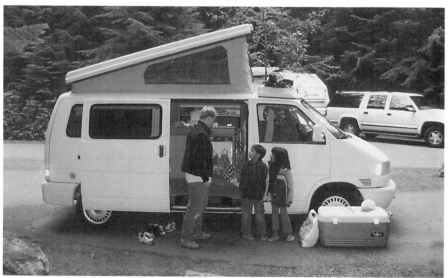

Who will get to sleep in the "upper berth" of this van?

camper. Vans are compact and easy to drive. Alaina's van has a pop-up top over a bunk where her kids, Oscar and Isabela, both 6, sleep. The kitchen and a double bed are on the main floor. Holly's EuroVan has a pop-up top with a bed, too, but her kids prefer to sleep in tents outside. When campers with a van arrive in camp, they park; no leveling is necessary. When it's time to leave, they secure the pop-up top and off they go.

Camper vans are expensive and hard to find. One dealer, who told me they no longer sell camper vans, told me that the last one they sold went for $44,000. I talked to Duane at a company near my home that is a "custom shop." They convert the van of your choice to a camper. Duane said that no two customers want the same things in their van, and that recent conversion costs ranged from $1500 to $15,000, depending on the amenities that were installed. He said that storage was the biggest concern of their customers.

Renting

As a novice camper, you may still be confused or at least undecided about which to choose among the many possibilities—tent, RV, or something in between. Remember, the good news is that you don't have to make a permanent decision when you're planning your first camping trip. If you want to begin by trying a tent, call up those

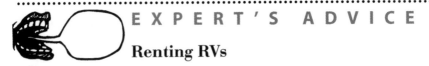

E X P E R T ' S   A D V I C E

Renting RVs

If you're thinking of renting an RV, Roger Arnell of RV Gold, Inc., recommends renting the smallest RV that can possibly meet all your needs for sleeping and safe travel. This will ensure that you're comfortable but not paying too much in rental fees or gas for an RV that is larger than you need.

friends who will let you borrow one. Better still would be friends who have more than one tent, and who would camp with you that very first time. If not, you can always rent a tent for your camping trial. Look in your local phone directory for rental companies and outdoor stores, and call around to see if they rent tents and other camping equipment. The REI store in my city rents tents, stoves, sleeping bags, pads, and lanterns. REI has outdoor stores all over the US; to find one close to you, call 800-426-4840 or go to www.rei.com.

C H E C K L I S T

Questions to Ask When You're Renting an RV

▶ How large of a unit do I need?

▶ What furnishings are included?

▶ How will I be charged?

▶ What about insurance?

▶ What happens in case of a breakdown?

If you want to begin by trying an RV, renting is even easier. Almost every city has RV rental agencies. If you can't find one where you live, you can drive or fly to a nearby city and pick up your RV there. Or you can have the RV delivered. Roger Arnell, of RV Gold Inc. near Sandy, Oregon, told me that most of his deliveries are to the airport in Portland or Seattle, but for a small fee he will also deliver to your home in Washington, Oregon, or northern California.

Roger recommends that you rent the smallest RV that can possibly meet all your needs for sleeping and safe traveling space. It will be easier to drive and also will use the least amount of fuel.

If you pick up the RV in your own city, you can drive it home and load it up with your own dishes, kitchenware, and bedding, but if you drive or fly to a pick-up destination, you may need to rent those necessities. Roger calls them "convenience kits." When Roberta and her family flew to Las Vegas to tour the national parks in a Cruise America rental, they paid extra for furnishings, but when Sara and her family flew to San Francisco to camp at Yosemite, they each checked two suitcases, one with city and camp clothes, and the other with camping equipment.

When you're making rental arrangements, be sure to factor in the cost of the furnishings that you will need. On the big island of Hawaii, two agencies rent camper trucks. At first glance, one seems much more expensive than the other. When you look close-ly at what you're getting, the cheaper rental is bare bones; any-thing you might need—bedding, cookware, dishes, beach umbrella, propane stove—is extra. On the other hand, the more expensive rental includes everything you might want for a week of Hawaiian camping.

There are some important questions to ask at the time that you rent: How will you be charged, by the day or by the miles? What is the fee if you drive extra miles beyond what is allotted? Will your automobile or homeowner's insurance policy cover you in the event of an accident, or do you need to buy additional insurance? What happens if you have a breakdown in the rented RV? Who should you call? Who pays for towing?

Resources for RV Renters and Buyers

If you're thinking of renting or buying an RV, there are many sources on the internet and in magazines to check for detailed information on driving and towing, shopping for a new or used RV, and comparing different units so you can find the best one for you.

The Good Sam Club, an organization of RV owners, is dedicated to making RVing safer and more enjoyable. They offer discounts, trip-routing, and other services, and in many areas they support local chapters for one-on-one advice and mentoring. They also have advice for RVing with children. Reach them at www.goodsamclub.com or 800-234-3450.

GoRVing (www.gorving.com), a service developed by RV dealers, will send you a free getting started video for first-time RVers. Another good site for sharing general RV information is www.rver-sonline.org. If you're worried about driving the RV, RV Rite (253-435-8666) sells training manuals for all recreation vehicles. Several magazines might also be helpful, including *Camping Life Magazine* (www.campinglife.com or 310-537-6322), *Motorhome Magazine* (www.motorhomemagazine.com or 800-678-1201), or *Trailer Life* (www.trailerlife.com or 800 825 6861). Some of these publications will send you one free issue or sign you up for an online newsletter. *Camping Life* plans to debut a television program on the Outdoor Life Network in 2006.

Where Shall We Go?

We live in a wonderful country. We have an unbelievable number of places to camp in the US. Planners or visionaries at every level of government, national, state, county, and even some cities, have provided sites where we can park our motorhomes or set up our tents. In some areas, it's possible to "camp" in a cabin, a yurt, or a refurbished caboose. And that's not counting private campgrounds or parks in Canada!

If you already know where you are going for your upcoming camping trip, you can skip this section and go on to the next. But maybe you've never ever camped before. Maybe you're not sure of where you want to go and you want some help finding a spot. Or perhaps you know what you want, a forest or a swimming lake or a place to fish, but you don't know where to find it. You might simply be overwhelmed by all the choices and don't know how to begin selecting a destination.

In any of those cases, stick with me. This section begins with a discussion of planning first camping trips, which will probably be close to home. The sections that follow describe public and private camping choices, and then

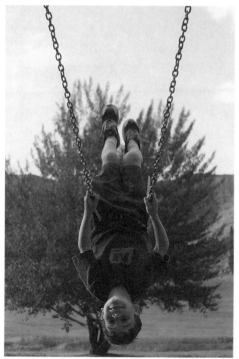

Some campgrounds have playgrounds.

camping farther afield. You will learn how to make and use an itinerary, how to research out-of-state campgrounds, and how to find private campgrounds. The last sections cover making reservations and camping without reservations.

How Much Travel Will Your Children Tolerate?

The most important guideline in all the planning that you do is knowing what your kids will tolerate. If this is a weekend trip—one day out, one or possibly two nights away, and one day to return—figure out how many hours your kids are willing and able to spend on the road in one day.

Janetta, a single mom, realized that she and her daughter could tolerate a drive of only one and a half hours from Seattle, singing and talking, while Jeanie and her husband were able to drive for three hours from their home in Bakersfield, California, to good fishing spots. Jeanie says she spent most of the drive reading to young Christine.

Don't assume that your kids will be sitting in the car the whole time you're driving; build into your trip the time for several stops where the kids can get out and run around. Plan for these stops in highway rest areas, in towns along the way where you can look for playgrounds in local parks or school grounds, or in fast food outlets that have play facilities attached.

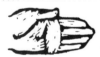

HELPING HANDS

The Destination Game

To determine where you should camp, first figure out how many hours of driving your family can tolerate. Next, enlist your children's help for this exercise: Using the distance key on the map, cut a piece of string that represents the distance you can travel from your hometown. Tie the string to a pencil. On a map of your state, pin the other end of the string over your hometown, and draw a circle as many hours away as your family can drive in one day. Your destination is somewhere in that circle. Look for the symbols for overnight camping.

First Camping Trips

After you decide on the number of hours your family can travel in one day, you can determine where you should go. Here is a simple trick to help you do this: First, get out a map of your state and, using the map's scale, measure a piece of string that represents the distance on the map your family is willing to travel. Next, tie one end of the string to a pencil and, with your finger, pin the other end on the map on your hometown. Now pull the string taut with the pencil and draw a circle around your hometown.

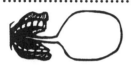

E X P E R T ' S   A D V I C E

Two Rules for First-Timers

1. Don't go too far from a town for your first effort, in case you forget something important.

2. Make your first trip short, even if you have a lot of time, until you get the hang of camping.

The circle's radius—the length of the string—represents the distance your kids can tolerate in the car to your campground. In other words, if your kids can tolerate only four hours of driving, the string will equal four hours' distance according to the scale of the map that you are using. Your destination is somewhere in that circle. Your older children can do the string test for you, and then look inside the circle for the little red tent or green tree that symbolizes overnight camping on the map.

You may be surprised to see how many opportunities for camping lie very close to your own home. I did a little test. I figured that a fussy child, or his parents, might not put up with more than one hour, or 50 miles, in a car. I drew a circle with a 50-mile radius from my home to see how many camping choices I have. Lots. Of course, lucky me, here in Seattle I can select from among saltwater beaches, freshwater lakes, lowland forests, or parks in the foothills of the Cascade Mountains. I have a choice of county parks, state parks, or national forests. Three national parks are just a little more than one hour away. And my map doesn't show private campgrounds, but in the yellow pages of my telephone book, I counted five entries for "Campgrounds" and 20 for "Recreational Vehicle Parks," all within 50 miles of my home.

In the April 2004 issue of *Parent Map*, a monthly newsmagazine for Seattle-area parents, Hilary Benson describes her family's first camping trip with sons ages 2 and 4. It was spent at a city-owned park in Seattle, only 10 minutes from home. They arrived at Camp Long in late afternoon, cooked and ate dinner outdoors, spent the night in sleeping bags in a cabin, breakfasted hastily the next morning, and left for home at 8:30 a.m. Fourteen hours altogether. A very good first campout.

Even if you have a whole week of vacation and not just a short weekend, for your first campout with small children you are better off planning a trip of only one or two nights until you get the hang of camping. A week may be too long for a first camping trip in a tent. Although a week in a motorhome or camper could be made bearable even if it rained every day, it wouldn't be fun. If you have a whole week for vacation, take your two-day trip in the middle of the week when parks and facilities are less crowded, and do other things before and after.

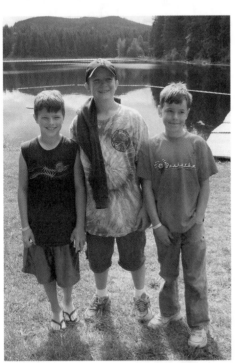

Happy campers are those who follow the two rules for first-timers (page 43).

Don't go too far from a town for your first effort, in case you forget something important. "Be close to a town that has food," Julia, 12, advised. She may be like my grandchildren, who as young teenagers preferred fast food in town to camp cooking. Eight-year-old Eliot's grandfather would agree on staying close to town; when we met the two of them in a US Forest Service camp outside of Seattle, he had forgotten one bag of their provisions and they had to drive back to go shopping.

My friend Barb told me about her family's first camping trip, a backpack of one week when her children were 5, 6, and 7. The hiking turned out to be much too arduous for the kids, they did not have enough waterproof clothing, and the tarp they slept under leaked water through the sides. They had to dry their socks over an open fire and ration their food because they hadn't packed enough. Nevertheless, they got through the week because, she said, her husband was so good and so patient with the children. And they weren't turned off from camping, but after that first trip they bought a real tent and revised their expectations of what their kids could do.

Public Camping Choices

Eliot, 8, and his grandfather, and Barb and her family, were camping in very primitive situations. In Eliot's Forest Service campground, the road was paved, but the pullouts for cars were gravel. The camping sites were spacious. There was one central pump for getting water, and there were outhouses scattered through the grounds. Barb's campsites were even more primitive; the toilets were boxes hidden discreetly in the brush, and water had to be pumped from a stream.

Many campgrounds in national and state parks are just like the one where Eliot was camping. Other more developed parks have paved roads and paved pull-outs for parking cars or RVs. They sometimes, but not always, have bathrooms with flush toilets and coin-operated showers. The RV sites have connections to electricity and water, and some have sewer connections also. Many parks that don't have sewer connections have a dumping station near the exit from the park. Some have pull-through sites so drivers won't have to back their motorhomes or trailers out of their spaces. Some restrict the

Quick Quiz

Who Runs the Campgrounds?

Q: Which government agencies in your neighborhood might administer camp-grounds?

A: National Park Service, US Forest Service, Bureau of Land Management, the state Park Service, the county Parks Department, or the city Parks Department.

Some people are surprised to find that even publicly owned campgrounds charge a daily fee. At Mt. Rainier National Park, which has five campgrounds, daily fees run from $8 to $15, depending on the park. Since they have no RV hook-ups, the cost is the same for tent or RV campers. The charge at Oregon State Parks runs from $13 to $18 per day for tent campsites during the high, summer season, and from $17 to $23 per day for full hook-ups. In addition, all campers in Oregon who make advance reservations pay a $6 nonrefundable reservation fee. At the Forest Service's primitive campgrounds (those with wooden outhouses and a central water tap) on I-90, an hour's drive from my house, the fee per day is $16 per campsite, but at remote campgrounds, miles of dirt roads away from highways, camping is free.

These fees are in addition to the fee that you pay when you enter the park, which may vary from park to park. If you take a grandparent with you when you camp at a national park or forest, you won't have to pay an entry fee if Grandma or Grandpa has a Golden Age Passport. This lifetime permit for anyone 62 or older gets the whole carload into the park free. You can buy the passport at ranger stations or some federal office buildings.

size of the RV to no longer than 25 feet. Those campgrounds that are run by governmental agencies—national, state, and county—usually are located close to some kind of natural attraction, like a lake, a river, or an area with lots of hiking.

When you're looking for a park, keep in mind some of the code words associated with campsites. "Primitive" or "undeveloped" sites have just a picnic table and a space for a tent; primitive parks have vault outhouses and no showers. They may have a centrally located water tap, or your water may come from a nearby stream. Parks that have "developed" sites have spaces with RV hook-ups that could be "full hook-ups," with water, electricity, and sewer, or "partial hook-ups," with just water and electricity. Many public parks have some combination of developed and undeveloped campsites. Some private

RV parks have cable, phone, internet access, and cable TV in addition to the usual hook-up. Ask about charges. Is water and electricity included in the overnight fee, or is there a separate meter for each of those? (For information about locating public campgrounds, see the section on Reservations, page 56.)

Private Camping Choices

Private campgrounds have many more amenities than public campgrounds. Their lawns are manicured, and they have flush toilets, showers and laundry facilities. In a KOA campground women's restroom, I saw a special tub for bathing babies. Private campgrounds usually include special recreational facilities, like a swimming pool or tennis courts, but there are not always natural attractions nearby.

Although they may have a few tent sites, more private campgrounds are set up for RVs. The better parks advertise pull-throughs. Other refinements may include cable TV and phone lines. One park described itself as "modem friendly." Some RV parks provide more electricity (more amps) than public campgrounds.

CHECKLIST

Questions to Ask About RV Parks

▶ What is the fee per night, and what does it include?

▶ Is there a restriction on the length of the RV?

▶ Does it have pull-throughs?

▶ How many amps does it provide for each space?

▶ Is there a laundry room and showers?

▶ Does it have telephone lines and cable TV?

▶ Is it modem-friendly?

▶ Is there a swimming pool?

If I can generalize from the descriptions I have collected, the private campgrounds are more luxurious than public parks, and they seem to provide more social activities, like swimming pools, playgrounds, or a meeting hall with evening movies and parties. The public parks seem less manicured, more natural, creating a greater sense of roughing it, being part of an unspoiled countryside. In public parks, you swim in a lake and attend a ranger's campfire talk in the evening.

In either kind of park, the campsites may be spacious, with hedges of greenery between one campsite and its next door neighbor, or they may be tiny with no separation between them at all.

Private campgrounds, as you might expect, are a little more expensive than public campgrounds. However, fees vary, with each owner setting his own. I checked the rates at some KOA camp grounds. On the coast of Washington, at Ilwaco, the daily fee ranges from $30 to $40 for an RV, and $26 to $36 for a tent. At a beach in California, the range is $37 to $57 for an RV, and $27 to $38 for a tent. Traveling inland, in Spokane, Washington, the fees range from $29 to $33 for an RV, and $24 to $27 for a tent, while in Needles, California, the rates are $22 to $32 for an RV and $19 to 20 for a tent. All these fees are for two people, and the rate charts say extra fees may apply for more people.

Yogi Bear's Jellystone Parks, another association of private camps, charges $20 to $40 per day for four people, with $5 per day per extra person over the age of 3.

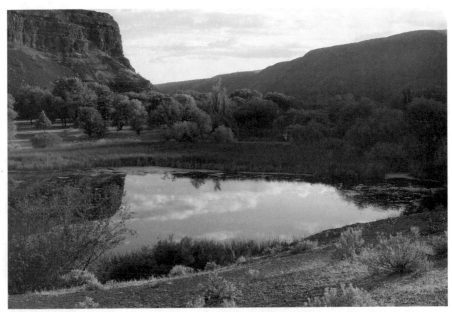

Many campgrounds are close to natural attractions.

Western Horizons Resorts, a membership organization, offers three or four nights complimentary camping to potential new members; all they ask is that you sit through a 90-minute promotional presentation. And if the campground isn't full, the manager may allow you to stay on at the regular rate. They have 22 resorts in 13 states.

Finding Private Campgrounds

While state publications list some private campgrounds, you can also find campgrounds by looking through the directories of those private campground organizations in this country and Canada that don't require a membership. (Keep in mind, however, that campers who buy a special card may receive a discount.) Kampgrounds of America, or KOA, with 475 locations, is the largest of these organizations. You can reach KOA by phone at 406-248-7444, or online at www.koa.com. Western Horizon Resorts (866-453-9305 or www.whresorts.com), has 22 camps located in seven western states,

Three Ways to Find a Private Campground

1. Contact a private campground chain such as KOA Kampgrounds (406-248-7444 or www.koa.com), or an association such as Jellystone Parks (800-558-2954 or www.campjellystone.com) or Western Horizon Resorts (866-453-9305 or www.whresorts.com).

2. Look in publications produced by Woodall's Publishing Corp.: 805-667-4100, 800-323-9076, or www.woodalls.com.

3. Check out RV shows and RV and camping magazines.

two southern states, two midwest states, and two east coast states. Yogi Bear's Jellystone Camps can be reached at www.campjellystone.com or 800-558-2954. I love their website, which includes a special section called "Just for Kids." Most of their camps are in the eastern and southern states, with only a few as far west as Colorado and Montana. While all these camps seem to be set up for RVers, they also have tent sites and many have cabins to rent as well.

Some privately owned campgrounds that are part of a membership network are also willing to accept nonmembers. Woodall's Publishing Corp. produces great directories for finding these campgrounds in the US and Canada. Contact Woodall's at 805-667-4100 or 800-323-9076, or visit www.woodalls.com. If you're looking for a camping experience with a minimum of preparation, the first part of one Woodall's catalogue, appropriately named *Go&Rent...Rent&Go*, lists private campgrounds that have at least three rental units on site, ready for you to move into (Go&Rent); these units could be RVs, trailers, tents, tepees, or cabins. The second part of that catalog is a directory of RV rental agencies (Rent&Go).

Magazines devoted to RVing and camping are also good resources for finding RV parks and campgrounds. *RVLife*, which covers RV camping in the Northwest, lists a number of campgrounds in its "Yellow Pages," and also has advertisements for campgrounds in the Northwest and beyond. *RVLife* is given away free at shows, but otherwise you have to buy single issues or subscribe. When you are attending RV shows, look for the free advertisements that might tell you where to go camping. National magazines on RVing and camping, such as *TrailerLife*, *Motorhome*, and *CampingLife*, will also help you find a private campground. (See Resources, page 242.)

Camping Farther Afield

When you're ready for a longer trip, use the same string technique for measuring the distance your family will travel in one day. If you're going to spend all your time in one place, your planning is the same. But if you propose to camp at more than one place, you have to build into your travel hours the time it takes to set up and break down your camp each day.

Another friend, Maggie, and her family camp for a week or more at a time. They move around, but they try to camp at no more than three different sites. If you have a camper or a motorhome, it's easier to move. Maggie's family camps in a tent, and she says it's a lot of trouble to put the tent up, take it down the next morning, and set it up again in a different place in the evening. Their camping trips tend to be triangular, so that they have a change of scenery, with at least two nights at each site. They may leave town driving in one direction, toward the coast, then veer away inland on their next leg, toward the mountains, and return on a different highway than the one they left on. You can do that in Washington State.

Make an Itinerary

When your plans involve moving from one park to another, it helps to make an itinerary, just like travel agents do for an extended tour. Write down where you will be on Day One, where you will spend the night, where you will go the next day, Day Two, where you will spend the night then, and so on.

Once your basic plan is determined, you can flesh it out with dates, meals and menus, and the number of hours it will take to

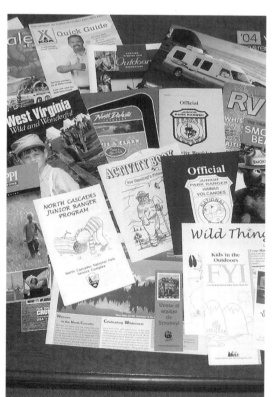

drive to each destination. Putting in the meals along the way (B for breakfast, L for Lunch, and D for dinner) will help you plan the numbers of meals you will need to pack. Then you can add a projected departure time for each day.

Whether you're camping in a tent or in an RV, be sure to allow time for breaking camp on each departure day and for a break in the middle of a long driving day. Once you've figured out your itinerary, you can make reservations.

Planning future trips? Create a camping resource library.

IMAGINARY CAMPING

One Week in the Pacific Northwest

Follow me on an imaginary weeklong camping trip. Saturday through the following Sunday, I'm going to leave Seattle and visit three different parks, camping in Olympic National Park in Washington, and then going on to Jesse M. Honeyman and Fort Stevens State Parks in Oregon. My itinerary would look something like this:

Day One: Drive from Seattle to Olympic National Park

▶ Leave 8 a.m., breakfast at home; lunch en route; dinner in camp.

▶ Stop in Port Angeles for lunch and a break.

▶ Overnight in Olympic National Park.

Day Two: Olympic National Park

▶ Breakfast, lunch, dinner in camp; overnight in park.

Day Three: Drive to Oregon Coast

▶ Leave ONP 10 a.m.; arrive Honeyman State Park 5 p.m.

▶ Breakfast in ONP; lunch en route; dinner in Honeyman State Park.

▶ Stop in Seaside, Oregon, for lunch and a break.

▶ Overnight in Honeyman State Park.

Keep your itinerary in hand when you are planning meals for the trip. Plan to use fresh foods early and turn to dried and canned foods later in the trip. Pack later meals at the bottom of your food containers and early ones on top. Or, if you plan to shop for fresh foods along the way, build those stops into your itinerary. (Read the sections What Do We Need?, page 61, and How Do We Cook in Camp?, page 153.)

Looking at the sample itinerary I have drawn, you can see that you will need to provide eight lunches, but only seven breakfasts and dinners—your first breakfast and last dinner will be eaten at home. Some of the lunches are en route. You can decide to pack those meals and picnic on the way, or you can stop in a restaurant.

Day Four: Honeyman Park

▶ Breakfast, lunch, dinner in camp; overnight in Honeyman Park.

Day Five: Honeyman Park

▶ Breakfast, lunch, dinner in camp; overnight in Honeyman Park.

Day Six: Drive to Fort Stevens State Park

▶ Leave Honeyman Park at 10 a.m.

▶ Breakfast at Honeyman Park; lunch en route; dinner at Fort Stevens.

▶ Stop in Lincoln City, Oregon, for lunch and a break.

▶ Overnight in Fort Stevens Park.

Day Seven: Fort Stevens State Park

▶ Breakfast, lunch, dinner in camp; overnight in Fort Stevens Park.

Day Eight: Return to Seattle

▶ Leave Fort Stevens 10 a.m.

▶ Breakfast in camp; lunch en route; dinner at home.

▶ Stop in Centralia, Washington, for lunch and a break.

▶ Arrive home at 5 p.m.

If you're camping in an RV, it's easy to pull over into a rest stop, eat lunch at a picnic table or inside, and then allow the children some running around time. If you're a tent camper, you can do the same, but it's a little more work to get the lunch fixings out and put away again. Some people would rather stop at a restaurant or fast food outlet, especially if it's the kind that has its own playground.

Researching Out-of-State Campgrounds

I know that all states are not as rich in camping opportunities as mine is, so I did some research on camping elsewhere. Since most of my camping has been done in Washington, Oregon, and

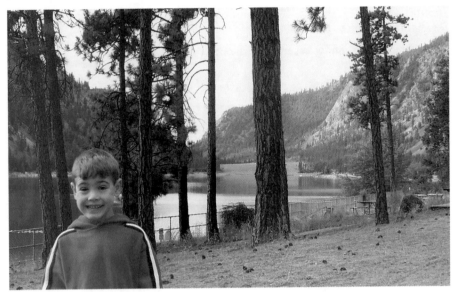

Think about your requirements for a campsite. Do you need one with a wonderful view?

California, I chose to investigate several other states that I did not know well. I purposely selected states that aren't particularly renowned camping destinations. Suppose you're visiting grandma in a faraway state and you plan to camp at interim stops on your way. You can research your journey the same way I did.

I used three methods for getting information. First, I called my directory assistance number and asked for an 800 number for tourism in Mississippi and West Virginia. I called those numbers and asked them to send me information about camping in their states. Then I wrote a brief, hand-written note asking for "information about camping in your state," and mailed it to "State Office of Tourism" in the capitals of North Dakota and Kansas. Last, I picked three states to contact online. I went to the websites for Nebraska, Rhode Island, and Ohio. On each site I was able to ask to have information about camping mailed to me.

Each of the states I queried replied in a timely manner, with a large packet of beautifully photographed booklets and brochures, including a good map. Tourism is big business, and states are eager to entice visitors by sending them lots of information about the attractions of their state and the accommodations of all kinds that are available.

For instance, Mississippi sent me a 214-page *Official Tour Guide*, a separate *Hunting, Fishing, and Outdoor Recreation* book, and a pamphlet on their 28 state parks.

North Dakota's travel guide has nine detailed pages on campgrounds listed alphabetically by nearest town. For instance, the capital, Bismarck, has four campgrounds nearby. Typical of the facts about each campground that all the states provided, the Bismarck KOA Campground, 1 mile north of town on I-94, Exit 161 (easy to find if I were in Bismarck), has 47 full hook-ups, 25 with only water and electric, four camping cabins, and also tent sites, showers, a pool, a dump, a central modem, laundry, playground, and tennis and basketball courts. It also has a website, an email address, and a phone number. It's almost more than you want to know!

Even little Rhode Island lists 35 camps on their website, some saltwater beach state parks, some forests, and some private campgrounds. (One is a nudist camp!) I learned that Rhode Island state parks have lower fees for residents than nonresidents.

Three Ways to Research Campgrounds in Another State

1. Call the 800-number for the tourism office in that state.
2. Write a letter addressed to the Tourism Office in the capital of the state.
3. Go online to the website of the state (every state has one).

Only Ohio neglected to include camping lore among all the material they sent, although their state map clearly shows state parks with an overnight camping symbol. It's important to emphasize, when you make your request, that you're interested in camping. Even more important, let them know that you will be camping with children, because some, but not all, states have special Junior Ranger programs for kids.

All the other states provided similar information. All of them have camping opportunities, both public and private, which are described in great detail: lakes for swimming, lakes for fishing, boat launching, hiking, proximity to historic places, and more.

Reservations

When Roberta and her family flew to Las Vegas to pick up an RV from Cruise America, a national RV rental company, for a tour of the national parks in the southwest, they not only had reserved spots at the campgrounds they were interested in, they had also reserved one night at an elegant Las Vegas resort at each end of their trip. Whether you choose a private campground or a state or national park, it's a good idea to call or write ahead or go online for a reservation.

If you're going to a well-known, popular campground, there is a risk to going without a reservation, especially on holiday weekends. Many parks fill up well in advance of the choicest days. Marlene makes her reservation just after midnight on New Year's Eve for Memorial Day weekend at a very popular park. Oregon State Parks takes reservations nine months in advance; when I talked to the

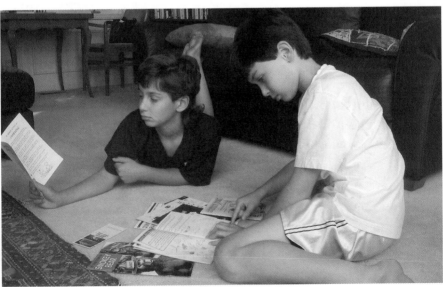

For some kids, researching campgrounds is serious business.

reservations clerk just before Labor Day, she was taking reservations for early June of the next year.

You can contact the National Park Reservation Service to make campground reservations at some but not all national parks up to five months in advance. That means that if you reach them on February 5, you can make reservations from February 6 to July 5. Make reservations at www.reservations.nps.gov, or call 800-365-2267.

• •

Four Great Resources
for Making Campground Reservations

1. National Park Reservation Service: www.reservations.nps.gov or 800-365-2267.

2. National Recreation Reservation Service: www.reserveusa.com or 877-444-6777 (TTY 877-833-6777 for the hearing impaired).

3. Reserve America: www.reserveamerica.com.

4. The phone numbers or internet addresses listed in the reference materials from state and regional tourism agencies.

• •

Another good resource for making online campground reservations at national facilities is www.reserveusa.com, the address of the National Recreation Reservation Service (NRRS), a one-stop reservation service for the US Forest Service, Army Corps of Engineers, National Park Service, Bureau of Land Management, and Bureau of Reclamation outdoor recreation facilities and activities. Their toll-free number is 877-444-6777 (for the hearing impaired, TTY 877-833-6777).

A related website, www.reserveamerica.com, includes some state parks as well as national facilities and private campgrounds. At this site, there is a list of phone numbers for reserving spots in some, but not all, states, but they don't have a general phone number. Or you can use the phone numbers or internet addresses in your reference materials to reserve a spot in the park in the state of your choice. Often when you go to the website for the park that you're interested in, you find a map of the campground and you can choose your very own site!

Be specific about what you're asking for. Two Rivers State Recreation Area in Venice, Nebraska (not far from Omaha), has only 10 caboose camping cabins but 90 tent sites and 83 sites for trailers. If you promise the kids a caboose, be sure that you have reserved one.

C H E C K L I S T

Questions to Ask When Reserving a Campsite

▶ Is the park available on the dates that I want?

▶ Where is the campsite located in the park? How far from the nearest bathroom/outhouse, water tap, beach?

▶ What kind of barrier, if any, is there between campsites?

▶ If I arrive in the park and I don't like my assigned site, can I move?

▶ Is there anything going on in the park—construction or other interruptions—that I should know about?

▶ How late can I arrive before I lose my reservation?

▶ How many nights can I stay in the park?

▶ What is the fee per night?

Ask about the cut-off hour for saving your reservation. At Jesse M. Honeyman State Park, a very popular park near Florence, Oregon, we arrived at 6:15 p.m. and found that our tent site next to the rest of the family had been given away at 6! Fortunately, other sites were still vacant. If you plan to stay at the same camp for more than one night, make your reservation for the full number of nights you want; some very popular state and national parks limit the length of time you can stay. Ask at the same time about the fees for the night; few campgrounds are free anymore.

The park may ask you to confirm your reservation with a credit card number, or, conversely, some smaller parks may not accept credit cards, so you will be expected to pay in cash when you arrive. Be prepared.

Although making a reservation on the web is certainly convenient, especially for people who work all day and do their planning late at night, I personally prefer to make arrangements by telephone, so I can ask questions about the park. Not that I would change my plans if I found out that there were no showers, or pit toilets instead of flush, but I don't like surprises. When I visited a Forest Service campground outside of Seattle that was supposed to have campsites accessible for the disabled, I found them no different from the others.

Also, I would want to know if there is anything going on in the park that isn't on the website, like construction or a beach closure. If I plan to camp outside of the summer season, either in early spring or late fall, I need to know if the campground is open. And I like to ask very specific questions about where the campsite is located in relation to the facilities of the park. Some park websites have maps that show this. If your computer isn't connected to your phone line, you can be looking at a map of the camp online while you are talking to the person who takes reservations.

Camping Without Reservations

Not all campgrounds accept reservations. Some national forest camps or small county parks, especially those where the plumbing is an outhouse and the water supply a tap, may not be set up with a reservation system. Or yours may not be the kind of family that makes reservations. Susan and her family like to be spontaneous, taking off without reservations when the urge strikes them, but they also never camp on weekends. Their work situations allow them to take their "weekends" Sunday through Tuesday, and Susan said they never have a problem getting into the campground of their choice.

If you decide to take off on the spur of the moment without a reservation, remember that it's first come, first served. You need to have a strategy for getting a good campsite. First of all, plan to arrive early in the day. Late in the day, there may be no sites left at all. Then

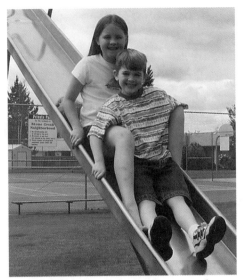

Some campgrounds have playgrounds with ball courts and jungle gyms for kids.

decide what is important to you. Do you need to be close to the outhouse, or to the lake? Is there a good level site for the tent? At many campgrounds, there is a designated pad for the tent; is this pad too small for your tent? Is the pad in good shape, level, and without a lot of twigs and stones? Maddy, 12, said that her family looks for shade and a nice place to have a fire, but her classmate Kate, also 12, tried to convince her family to leave a "creepy looking" site surrounded by so many trees no sunlight could get through.

Sara, an adult who finds camping a spiritual experience, wants her campsite to have a wonderful view, of mountains or a meadow or a lake. Diana's family likes the kind of campsite where you have to walk in a ways from the parking spot; it's a nuisance to carry all their equipment back and forth and it's farther from the bathrooms, but the quiet and privacy are worth it. Eight-year-old Eliot would agree; he told me that he and his grandpa had a wonderful campsite, with lots of land around it, because there was no one camped on either side.

You have to be flexible when you're choosing your campsite. On one trip, Diana and Larry found that the tent pad at their reserved campsite was in bad shape, the ground uneven and rocky. The parking area for the car was in much better condition, hard-packed and level and with fewer lumps, so they moved their car closer to the road and set up the tent at the end of the parking strip.

Our family always drove through the camping loops, looking over the empty campsites while we decide which one we like. Because we are tent campers, we try to avoid camping next to an RV, which might have annoying electrical features like bright lights, TV sets, or noisy generators. If the campground is popular and we see a likely looking site, we leave one of the older people in the group sitting at the picnic table while the rest of us continue to check out the other possibilities.

Summing Up

As I page through all the information that I have assembled, I imagine that my children are still young and I am planning a camping trip for my family. I have a list of campgrounds; I know the closest town to each. I know whether each park has RV hookups and/or tent sites or if I can rent a facility at that camp. There is a list of activities and amenities available at each park. All provide a telephone number for more information or for reservations, and some also include a website address.

I look through my guides. I think about my children's endurance, their tolerance for automobile trips. I find the areas within that parameter and look over the camps that are available to me. I see a lake, a forest, an historic site. Would the children like that? Would the adults in the family? Or maybe I first decide on the area I'd like to visit, and I check out the camps nearby. I see in the list of events taking place in that state that there is a festival in a nearby town on the weekend I'd like to visit. Would the children like that? Lots of choices. I can opt for only a weekend away, or plan to spend a whole week at the park of my choice, or design a route for a week or two of moving from camp to camp.

I make one decision, and now I have to make another: Should I pick up the phone or go to my computer to make my reservations?

What Do We Need?

When Susan and Bill's family decides to go camping, they all start piling the things they think they will need near the front door. They don't use a list or a system at all. They are experienced campers and they have a general idea of what they will need. If they forget something, and they always do, it just makes the trip that much more challenging and exciting. Once they forgot a warm jacket for one of their kids, and they formed a makeshift wrap for her out of some bedding. You may not want to camp like that.

While many of the kids I talked to were vague about how it was done, most of the grown-up campers had some kind of system for planning and preparing for camping. Most of the job was Mom's and much of the time it began with a list. Madelaine keeps a list on her computer where she can update it often. Marlene keeps a list in the garage with all her camping supplies; as soon as she comes home from one trip, she cleans her gear and gets it ready for the next one, changing the list as necessary. Ellen's RV is almost always ready to go.

CHECKLIST

Six General Categories of What You Need for Camping

▶ Shelter

▶ Sleeping

▶ Meals

▶ Clothing

▶ Fun

▶ Miscellaneous Gear for Comfort, Safety, First Aid, Repairs

I don't have a permanent list, but a week or so before I know we're going to go camping, I start jotting down the things we will need. I divide my list into six categories, which I also use in this section. We will need shelter, of course; sleep furnishings; meals (a camp kitchen as well as the food); clothing; stuff for fun; and a miscellaneous group of things like comfort, safety, repair, and first-aid items. This section also includes a discussion on packing and storage.

The ideas that follow include some suggestions from other campers that I would never use, just as they would not take everything on my list. The recommendations are meant to get you started on a list of your own. The list came from tent campers and RV campers alike; it was surprising to see how both groups make use of many of the same items. Don't be put off by thinking that the basics will require an investment of hundreds of dollars. Remember that many of the camping-specific items can be rented, borrowed, or found at garage sales, and other items, like clothing and kitchenware, you already own.

What You Need for Shelter

If you're camping in an RV, your vehicle is at the top of your list for planning and preparation. If you own the vehicle, you need to make sure that all the systems are working, and that all the tanks are in proper order. That means the fuel and water tanks are full and the waste tank is empty. If you're renting or borrowing the RV, you need to be doubly sure that whoever drove it last left it in good condition. Some RV campers also carry a tent, so they can take turns sleeping out of doors.

The basic list for tent campers starts, of course, with a tent, including its poles, stakes, ground cloth, and rain fly. You need tent stakes even if your tent is self-supporting, to keep it from blowing away. The ground cloth is a large piece of plastic spread under the tent to keep moisture from seeping up and to save the tent floor from wear and tear by small pebbles and twigs on the ground. A rain fly is a large tarp, often plastic, that can be set up over the picnic table and cooking area to keep it dry. Madelaine brings huge

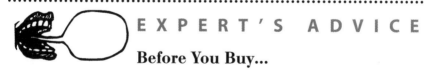

EXPERT'S ADVICE

Before You Buy...

When taking stock of what you need for camping, remember that many of these items can be rented, borrowed, or found at garage sales. Some items, such as clothing and kitchenware, you probably already own.

tarps and lots of ropes to rig as rain flies. They never let the rain drive them home, she said; instead, they try to find a campsite with lots of trees for attaching their tarps. You may also want to include a small broom to sweep out your tent before you pack it up.

Often, both RV campers and tent campers will set up comfortable folding chairs and loungers around their campsite. Holly told me that folding chairs have improved tremendously in recent years; she now owns a model with a very comfortable foot rest. Randy also brings a small folding chair for his daughter; he said it wasn't fair for the grown-ups to sit around the fire in their own chairs while Allie, 6, didn't have one. Maggie takes folding lawn chairs and grass mats for lounging.

C H E C K L I S T

Sheltering in a Tent

▶ Tent
▶ Tent poles
▶ Tent stakes (Do you have enough?)
▶ Rain fly
▶ Ground cloth
▶ Folding lawn chairs (optional)
▶ Screen house or sun shade (optional)
▶ Portable potty (optional)
▶ Broom (optional)

Some campers carry a screen house, which sets up like a tent but has only screen walls. These little screened rooms provide refuge from mosquitoes or other flying pests. In mosquito country, you sometimes see infants in their infant seats in the screen room while their older siblings are running around outside.

Other campers carry a sun or rain roof that also sets up like a tent but has no walls at all; these have various names, like canopy, sunshade, umbrella, gazebo, or arbor. You see these in campgrounds with no shade.

My favorite source for finding tents or sun shelters is the Campmor catalogue, which not only lists a wide variety of nationally known brands of tents and tent accessories, but also often carries these items at sale prices. Order a copy of the Campmor catalogue by calling 800-226-7667 or visiting www.campmor.com. When you buy or rent your canopy, make sure that stakes and guy ropes, if necessary, are included.

A portable potty is another good item for tent campers with small children. In the middle of the night when one of the kids wakes up and has to go, the park's bathroom may be far from your campsite, or the outhouse may be dark and scary for a child. A portable potty, set discreetly behind your tent or privately in a separate room, is close, safe, and familiar. In Utah, my daughter Judy found the collapsible cardboard Happy Seat, and on the web I found a couple of other versions of lightweight folding potties. (For more information, see Resources, page 242.)

When you pack the car, load the tent last so it can come out and be set up first. Be sure your tent is complete before you leave home. On one trip, Sandy and Pat forgot their poles, so they rigged up a kind of lean-to by tying the tent to the table and some trees, and they slept under that. They never forgot the poles again.

What You Need for Sleeping

When you're camping, you'll need something warm to sleep in. Sleeping bags are standard in tents and in some RVs. Kids like them, but if you're just getting started and you're not sure you want to invest in one, you can rig a warm nest of blankets and sheets.

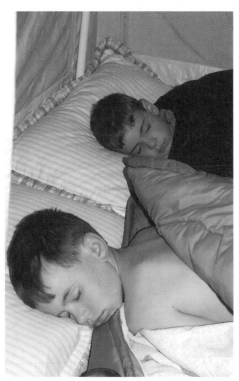

Don't forget good pillows!

Old blankets are a useful material for making sleeping bags. A single-bed-sized blanket or comforter folded in half and stitched together on two sides becomes a neat sleeping envelope.

Sleeping bags come in two shapes, the mummy bag, which is tapered at the foot, and the rectangular bag. Many people find mummy bags too restricting; if you're the kind of sleeper who thrashes around a lot at night, you'll be more comfortable in a rectangular bag. Mummy bags, which require more skillful construction, are generally more expensive than rectangular bags. Sleeping bags can range in price from under $20 to hundreds of dollars, depending on their intended use. The most expensive ones are designed for winter camping or climbers who spend the night on frigid glaciers; camping families don't need that kind.

CHECKLIST

What You Need for Sleeping

▶ A sleeping bag for every member of the family.

▶ Some kind of insulation under every sleeping bag.

▶ Some kind of padding for everyone who needs it .

The other factors affecting the price of the bags are the insulating materials and the covers. Goose down, which is very lightweight and very warm, is preferred by many backpackers. The disadvantage of down is that it loses its insulating qualities if it gets wet. Duck down is a little less expensive, but also not effective when wet. Down bags are generally covered with ripstop nylon or other very lightweight material, while other bags are covered with taffeta or cotton. Less costly synthetic materials like Polarguard or Hollofil are heavier than down but stay warm while wet, an important consideration if you have kids who may occasionally wet the bed. Sleeping bags intended for use in cabins or RVs or for warm nights are made of fleece.

I own three sleeping bags. The oldest, goose down covered with ripstop nylon, is for backpacking in the mountains. It has a hood that I can pull tight around my face on very cold nights so that only my nose sticks out. My second bag, a big and bulky rectangle, with nylon taffeta on the outside, polyester-fiber insulation, and cotton-flannel lining, is for car camping; the full-length zipper on this bag makes it possible to zip up with my husband's bag for a warm and cozy night. The third bag I made myself for a raft trip down the Colorado River in the Grand Canyon. I sewed three sides of a length of lightweight fleece to a single bed sheet to make a big double bag. Most nights were warm enough to sleep with the fleece on the bottom and the sheet over us, but on one cool night, we slept with the fleece on top.

Fleece is a wonderful material to work with. It doesn't ravel or fray, so the edges don't take special handling. If you make bags of fleece for your kids, they will have the added advantage of drying quickly if your child doesn't make it to the potty in a timely way. Fleece comes in several weights; be sure the fabric you buy will be warm enough for the area you're visiting.

When you shop for a bag, consider the night temperatures of the area where you'll be camping. Nights can be cool in the mountains and by the ocean, but inland camps are often warm. If you're going to be camping next to your car, you don't have to worry about the weight of the bag. If you're camping in a tent, you can expect to be colder than the family in some kind of RV. Inexpensive, warm but

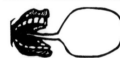

E X P E R T ' S   A D V I C E
Make Your Own Sleeping Bag

To make your own sleeping bag, fold an old comforter or a blanket in half and stitch it closed on two sides. You can make shorter sleeping bags for your kids in the same way; buy a length of fleece at a fabric store, fold it in half, and sew it up.

heavy sleeping bags can often be found in outlet stores or hardware stores; many outdoors stores geared toward serious mountaineers carry pricier goods.

Mattresses or sleeping pads or cots are more important for parents than for kids, who don't seem to suffer as much from sleeping on the hard floor. An air mattress cushions the sleeper from the hard floor of the tent and the little irregularities that stick up through it, but if the floor is cold, the air mattress will conduct body heat away from the sleeper into the floor. A closed cell foam pad is good insulation from the cold floor, but not as comfortable as an air mattress.

There was a time when I used both, the foam pad on the floor for insulation and the air mattress on top of it for comfort. Then I acquired a mat that is both padding and insulation, and on top of that it is also self-inflating. Mine is a brand called Therm-a-Rest, but several other labels make a variety of styles of camping mattresses and pads that also offer padding and insulation and are self-inflating. Some are quilted, some have ridges. There are also foam pads and air mattresses that have to be blown up, but you can use a pump to do that job.

For the person who really doesn't care to sleep on the tent floor, there are camping cots with metal or wooden frames that fit inside a tent. Some are only 8 or 9 inches high. These cots could be used with a sleeping bag or made up with regular bedding.

Kids have no trouble sleeping on the tent floor so long as it's not cold. A closed-cell foam pad will block out the cold, but so will an inch or two of folded newspaper, and you can use the newspaper as a fire starter in the morning. If you have a mat that you take to an exercise class, one of the kids can sleep on that.

RV campers may choose to sleep in sleeping bags too, or if your RV has regular mattresses, you can just make up the beds with the bedding in your linen closet. Remember, though, that it may be colder in your RV bed than it is in your bed at home. Wendy suggests an extra blanket for each bed, even if your RV is furnished with sleeping bags. Or you can turn on the furnace, if your RV has one, but be sure to allow for fresh air to come in.

What You Need for Meals

You're probably looking forward to all the delicious meals you will cook and eat in camp. Before you can cook the food, however, you have to get it to camp—dry foods dry, and perishable foods safe. When you're planning your trip, think about cooking gear, pots and pans, and a stove. Then you can think about food. (For information on how to set up a kitchen and cook in camp, see pages 136 and 153.)

Refrigerators and Coolers

Some RVs have refrigerators and freezers that have three different controls: They run on electricity when they are plugged in at a park with full hook-ups; they run on batteries while they are on the road; and when they are parked somewhere with no electric plug, they run on propane. RV campers assured me that switching from one to the other is just that, a simple switch.

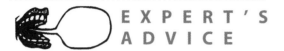

E X P E R T ' S A D V I C E

A Cool Idea

Consider Madelaine's solution for keeping food cold when camping: She freezes water in clean plastic milk jugs and uses them to keep her cooler cold. The ice melts but doesn't escape into the cooler, and that water can later be used for cooking.

Tent campers or those with less sophisticated RVs need some sort of icebox or cooler. Ice in the cooler melts and must be replaced periodically on a longer trip, so keeping food cold and getting rid of the water that collects in the cooler is a challenge. Often there are stores near a campground, or sometimes in the campground, which sell ice. Many metal insulated coolers have a spigot on the side that draws off most of the meltdown. Styrofoam coolers are cheaper to buy, but most must be emptied by tipping them up on their sides.

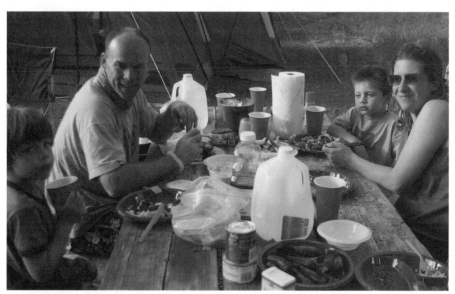

Food always tastes better outdoors.

C H E C K L I S T

What You Need for Meals

Food

▶ Storage containers

▶ Cooler and ice

▶ Supplies for breakfasts, lunches, and dinners

Cooking Tools

▶ Can opener

▶ Oven mitts

▶ Knife and cutting board

▶ Vegetable brush

▶ Tongs, spatula, fork

Items for Cleanup

▶ Dish pan

▶ Dish detergent

▶ Scouring pads

▶ Garbage bags

Kitchen Equipment

▶ Stove

▶ Fuel and matches

▶ Saucepans

▶ Teakettle

▶ Water carrier

▶ Dishes and flatware

Fire Pit Necessities

▶ Wood or charcoal

▶ Kindling

▶ Newspaper

▶ Bucket and shovel

▶ Spray bottle of water

Fire Pit Tools

▶ Grill

▶ Foil

▶ Hot-dog forks

▶ Marshmallow sticks

▶ Long-handled fork, tongs, spatula

The meal planners I talked to had many ingenious ways of taking care of these problems. Maggie arranges her foods in layers, first night on top. Meats or any other foods that would be hurt by soaking are carefully wrapped and enclosed in plastic bags. Foods for a second or third night out that would not be harmed by being frozen are frozen hard to help keep the cooler cold. Frozen fruit juices also help keep the cooler cold. Meals for a fourth or later night do not depend on foods from the cooler; instead she plans pasta with bottled sauce or replenishes her food and ice supply from stores near the campground. Susan reminded her that a solid block of ice will last longer than ice cubes.

Madelaine freezes water in clean plastic milk jugs and uses them to keep her cooler cold. The ice melts but doesn't escape into the cooler, and that water can later be used for cooking. She fills the jugs only halfway; water expands as it freezes and could break the jug if she filled it too full. Of course, artificial ice, plastic-covered compounds that freeze solid in a home freezer, will melt and not run at all, but there is no way of re-freezing them in camp once they thaw.

Many families take more than one cooler. They keep one handy in the car with juice, soft drinks, fruit, or other perishable snacks

IMAGINARY CAMPING
Moving the Kitchen Outside

As you go about preparing meals at home, think about the tools you would need if you were cooking in camp. Make a list of these items and adapt them to fit a camp kitchen. Perhaps some tools can be used for more than one purpose, to help you conserve space.

for consuming on the road. That way, the other cooler, which contains meats or eggs or dairy products, needn't be opened so often.

As coolers age, they tend to get smelly. An internet source suggests wiping the inside of the cooler with a very light application of vanilla after it has been cleaned. It must be real vanilla and not imitation. We usually leave our cooler outdoors in the sun on a hot day after it has been cleaned, and we always tilt the lid open when we store it.

Cooking Gear

Your cooking gear will depend on your menus. Here, again, you should practice imaginary camping. As you go about preparing meals at home, think about the tools you would need if you were cooking on a campfire or a camp stove. If you're heating canned soup for lunch, think can opener and sauce pan. If you're having one of those soups in a Styrofoam cup that you reconstitute with hot water, think of a kettle for boiling water.

Think through all the meals in your menu and imagine preparing them. If you're broiling steaks, you'll need a long-handled fork or tongs for turning them; if you're broiling hamburgers, you'll need a different tool for flipping, a long-handled spatula. Many fire pits in many campgrounds have an iron grill in place at the fire pit, but if you're not sure about what you will find in your camp, you can bring your own grill to place on the fire.

No grill? We set two or three tuna cans with both ends cut out in our campfire to hold our heavy iron frying pan. (I was impressed by the number of people who told me that they own heavy cast-iron pans and large kettles, just for cooking on the fire.) Also useful if you plan to make a campfire is a spray bottle of water to put out flames or sparks and a shovel or other tool to manage the fire.

Camp Stove

Though you may be planning to camp in an RV with a stove, oven, and microwave, many RVers also like to cook some of their meals outside, on a stove or on the campfire, just like the tent campers. So everyone should include a stove, fuel supply, and matches, as well as long-handled utensils for cooking on the fire (a pair of tongs, a spatula, a fork), in addition to the pots, pans, and the kettle for boiling water. Take a stove, even if you plan to do all your cooking on the fire pit. Sometimes, when the weather has been extremely dry, there is a ban on open fires; at other times, the wood may be wet and refuse to ignite.

Camp stoves use two kinds of fuel, white gas or propane. If your fuel is white gas, you'll need a funnel to refill the tank from your gas supply. If yours is a propane stove, take an extra cartridge. Be sure to read the instructions with either kind of stove carefully so you know how to light it and how to refuel. It's better to learn ahead of time how everything works, so you don't have problems when you're camping.

Wherever your kitchen may be, indoors or out, you will also need oven mitts for handling hot pans or foil packets, a sharp knife (with its tip in a cork for travel), a cutting board, a vegetable brush, and that can opener.

Fun Foods

Some of the tools for your kitchen are for fun foods. When I visited the classes at Assumption St. Bridget School, I learned about a campfire cooking gadget, a pie iron, which goes by various other names, too, like sandwich iron; Jack called it a "hobo iron." It gets used for lunch or snacks or dinner. Two iron cups on long handles close around two slices of bread with a filling in between. You clamp the sides together and hold it in the fire. As the bread toasts, the filling heats and melts.

All in the interest of scientific investigation, my husband bought a pie iron in a local outdoor store. Ours is called Coghlan's Camp Cooker (for more information, see Resources, page 242). We lunched on toasted sandwiches for several days, using the pie iron on our gas-fired barbecue. It was a lot of fun! We had all sorts of combinations, including peanut butter with a chocolate bar.

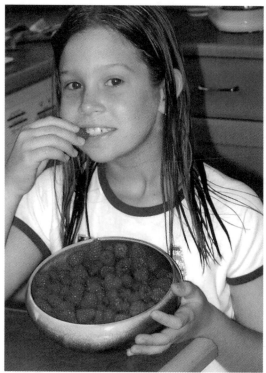

Other fun foods, and foods that children can cook themselves with some supervision, are hot dogs and s'mores. You'll need hot-dog forks and marshmallow sticks for these. Don't count on finding usable sticks in camp, and certainly don't plan to cut living plants for sticks.

Foil packet stew is another camp favorite in many families. If that's what you're having, be sure to pack heavy-duty aluminum foil and a long-handled tongs for

Fresh fruit is an easy fun food.

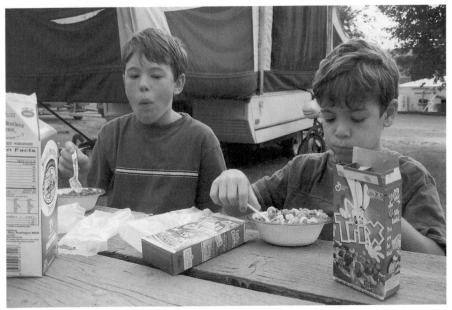

Cereal is still the breakfast of champions for campers.

getting the packets in and out of the fire. If you will be cooking pasta, bring a pierced spoon to lift it out of the boiling water.

A Dutch oven is another campfire cooking favorite in some families. A Dutch oven is a very heavy pot that sits in the coals and bakes delicious stews and desserts; think of it as a campfire slow cooker. The Dutch oven usually has three legs, to hold it above the coals, and a slightly domed lid that has a handle in the middle and a flange all around the edge. More coals are piled on top of the lid so the contents of the Dutch oven is heated from above and below. If you're using a Dutch oven, you should also have some kind of tool for grasping and removing the lid, and good-quality oven mittens. Dutch ovens can be stacked one on top of the other, biggest on the bottom, so several courses can cook at the same time.

If you hope to have a campfire, you should bring firewood from home, unless you are positive that it will be sold at the camp. Beware: Often the wood for sale in campgrounds is more expensive than wood brought in from outside. Again, don't expect to find wood to burn in camp. Except for little twigs, a campground will have been picked clean. While I was walking through a campground talking to campers with children, I noticed some people using fire logs in their campfires. They told me that these logs, made of compressed sawdust and wax, actually burn with less smoke and less ash than regular firewood. Some companies sell logs specifically designed for outdoor burning.

Whatever wood you bring, it should be of varying sizes. You don't start with the logs that give you a long-lasting fire. You start with newspapers and small sticks, kindling, and build up to the logs. You should bring plenty of newspaper for starting the fire, and a bucket and shovel for dousing that fire. In addition, a spray bottle of water is handy for dousing little flare-ups under your steak or hamburger.

Tableware

Eating gear, also depending on your menus, should include an unbreakable cup, plate, bowl, knife, fork and spoon for each member of the family, or, if you're going for disposables, enough plastic tableware and paper goods for every meal for each member of the family. Randy took his daughter shopping at an outdoor store so she could choose her own enamel dinnerware, which they use only for camping. Jane has a set of old Melmac plastic dishes for camping. A thrift store would be a good place to look for camping tableware.

A vinyl tablecloth or two dresses up your campsite and makes the table a little cleaner. Ruth recommends clips to fasten the tablecloth to the edge of the table, so it won't blow all over the foods.

Storage and Cleanup

Covers for food trays, often made of screening material, will keep flies and bees out of your food. You need at least one icebox or cooler for foods that are perishable, and another container with tight closure for foods that are not.

For cleanup after meals, you need one or two dish pans, with dish detergent and a scouring pad, a big box of plastic garbage bags, and possibly dish towels.

Water

If you are camping in a tent or if you didn't get a full hook-up for your RV, you'll need a water carrier to bring water from the central source to your site. If your water is taken from a stream or lake, you need to have a pump with a filter or else you need to treat it to make the water potable. In the US, potential contaminants of greatest concern are *Giardia lamblia* and *cryptosporidium*, both protozoa, and quite large, microscopically speaking, so a filter should catch them all. You can also boil water, which

> ## Quick Quiz
>
> ### Safe Water
>
> **Q:** How can you treat water that comes from a lake or stream?
>
> **A:** Boil it, filter it, or treat it with iodine. If you mask the taste of iodine-treated water with an electrolyte additive like Gatorade, you'll be taking care of two problems at the same time.

requires extra fuel for your stove, or you can use iodine tablets, which impart a funny taste to the water. Pumps, filters, and iodine systems are all available in outdoor stores. Lemonade mix can mask the taste of iodine-treated water.

The Food

Almost every one of the students who wrote an essay for me on camping commented on the food. Almost all of them had a favorite camp food, and even those who had had a mishap with food had learned from the experience. Even those students who wrote negatively about camping in general had positive things to say about camp food. Maybe it's true that food always tastes better outdoors, or maybe we're all just a little bit hungrier after a day spent in the open.

Although food was very important to them, the kids seemed almost unaware of a plan for meals in camp. Zach commented that the meals in their RV were just the same as what they ate at home. The moms, on the other hand, were unanimous in describing their meticulous meal planning. Susan brings food from home but does much of her shopping for fresh items in stores just outside the campground; she buys the best fruits and vegetables that are available. Madelaine hates shopping midway through a camping trip; she leaves home with two complete days of fresh food, and carries non-perishable canned goods for later days. Jeanie packs a food bag for each day; she flattens cooked casseroles, stews, and roasts in plastic bags in the freezer so they will fit in the ice chest. Holly pre-measures the ingredients of all the dishes she plans to cook in camp, and packages each dish together in one plastic bag. Wendy never takes boxes; she repackages all boxed food in zipped-up plastic bags so they take up less room.

When you pack, you need to double check to be sure you have all the ingredients for all the meals you plan to cook in camp, plus some snacks, plus extras, because appetites are often heartier in the outdoors. Use the itinerary you made to count the number of

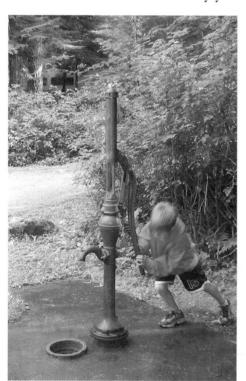

each kind of meal—breakfast, lunch, and dinner—that you will prepare. Don't forget tea bags and coffee for yourself when you're assembling drinks for your kids. Again, be an imaginary camper; if you're going to be using the pie iron, you need butter or non-stick cooking spray to coat the outside of the sandwich.

Is this a good time to try out new foods? The jury is out. Some parents say that "camping food" is special, not eaten at home or at other times, and therefore the unfamiliar is more readily accepted. Others

Pumping water takes strong muscles.

report just the opposite, that their children are unhappy over anything new.

Be sure to include snacks. Bridgit, who camps in an RV with two daughters under 5, keeps a variety of snacks together in one box—small boxes of raisins, trail mix, cookies, nuts, chips—so they don't tire of one kind.

Non-perishables need to travel in a separate container from the meats and eggs. Some campers use just the paper bags or boxes from the grocery store. Others own more permanent plastic boxes with snap-on lids or laundry baskets. Jane keeps her laundry basket ready to go with dishes, tableware, and non-perishable foods like canned soups and packaged noodles.

Once you're in camp, however, you must store attractive non-perishables somewhere safe from animals. Some campgrounds provide animal-proof lockers and require that you store all foods and scented toiletries in these so the products don't attract bears. If the campground doesn't provide lockers, you can store your food in the trunk or back of your car, or in a bag hanging from a tree limb. Hanging food from a tree is a fun task that kids can help with. Be sure to bring a sturdy bag and a long rope.

For a long and much more detailed consideration of foods for camping, see the section How Do We Cook in Camp, page 153.

What You Need for Clothing

Everyone in the family should have enough clothing, including swimsuits, sleeping clothes, warm jackets for evenings, and rain gear. Wendy likes a jacket with a zip-out lining, so she can adjust her layers according to the temperature. Everyone should have at least two pairs of shoes, one sturdy pair for hiking and another pair that can get wet. If you're buying new hiking boots for your vacation, break them in before you leave by wearing them around the house. (Some stores will allow you to return shoes if they haven't been worn outdoors.) My son Jeff added to this clothing list, extra socks. My friend Sandra recommended taking hats—a sun hat for warm days and a warm hat for cold nights.

Don't try to keep everyone spanking clean. Camping is roughing it, so an older shirt with a smudge or a stain is still an acceptable outfit. If a dirty shirt bothers you, you can turn it inside out and no one will see the dirt. You should have a variety of lightweight shirts for when it's really hot and warmer shirts to layer over them if the weather turns chilly.

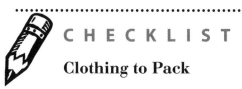

CHECKLIST

Clothing to Pack

▶ Swimsuit

▶ Sleepwear

▶ Warm jacket

▶ Rainwear

▶ Shoes and socks

▶ Sun hat and warm hat

▶ Everyday outfits, including underwear

Dress your children in bright colors, so you will be able to find them from a distance. Neutral colors are harder to see; a child in a green shirt in the woods will blend into the background colors more easily than the child in bright pink or orange. Cotton absorbs water and doesn't dry quickly; people dressed in cotton, caught in a rain storm, chill very rapidly. Some of the synthetics, like polyester, dry quickly and stay warm even when wet.

Here's how one family who camp in an RV plans their clothing: They count on one outfit per day, plus one extra. Daytimes are scruffy times when no one tries to stay clean. After their evening shower, however, the kids are changed into a clean outfit, and in the evenings they stay relatively clean. The next morning, the kids wear the same clean clothes they put on the night before. Their wardrobe includes a variety of clothing, long- as well as short-sleeved shirts, long pants and shorts, lightweight sweaters or sweatshirts, and one warm jacket. They pack appropriate numbers of underwear and socks. They always change into a clean outfit for the trip home.

Other families pack more or less than that. Those who have children who are recently toilet trained pack more underwear and shorts, because some kids forget their training in a strange situation. Some families pack less: At minimum, they have the one outfit they arrive in and one spare outfit to wear just in case the first one somehow gets soaking wet. They come home pretty raunchy.

Backpackers take scarcely any clothes at all. They wear the same things day after day, sometimes rinsing a garment out at night if they're certain it will dry by the next day. At Portland Luggage Company, I saw ultra-light socks and underwear that are supposed to dry rapidly. The store also carried disposable underwear that is supposed to withstand one washing. When I backpack, I change into polypropylene underwear in early evening so my day clothes can air, sleep in the underwear, and dress in the freshened day clothes the next morning.

Don't take your newest or best clothes camping. The warm jacket

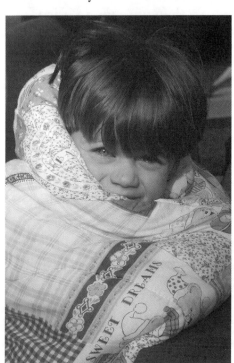

can be last year's almost outgrown school jacket. Bridgit has gone through her daughters' closets, pulling out the clothes that are no longer good enough for school, and packed them into boxes in their RV. That way, they're always ready for any kind of weather.

Camping is hard on shoes. The runners I wore in Hawaii last year are still stained red from walking on a muddy road. On the other hand, don't take your oldest, most worn shoes either. Choose a pair that has good tread left for walking. If you plan to

Pack a warm blanket to keep small campers snug.

buy new school shoes for your kids in September, take last year's on your camping trip. Each child should have a pair of sandals or flip-flops to wear for wading or into the shower.

If it rains, everyone will need effective rain gear. A big garbage bag can be used as a temporary raincoat if you forgot to pack one. Make a garment by cutting a hole in the top for the head and a hole on each side for the arms. Don't do this with really young children who might not understand the danger of pulling an uncut plastic bag over their heads.

Whether you pack everyone's clothes together or give everyone in the family some kind of container of their own (more about packing later), you need to plan for dirty clothes, with a common big laundry bag or individual bags. Madelaine adds a common bag for all the shoes.

What You Need for Fun

A camera is fun, and so are toys, but too many extras can become a nuisance. Bicycles, scooters, skateboards, roller skates, and tricycles all appear in camp. You also see Whiffle balls and

 C H E C K L I S T

Things to Bring for Fun

Wheeled Toys
▶ Bicycles
▶ Scooters
▶ Skateboards
▶ Skates

Beach Toys
▶ Shovels
▶ Dump trucks
▶ Air mattresses and water toys

Active Games
▶ Bat and balls
▶ Badminton set
▶ Frisbees
▶ Croquet set

Quiet Times
▶ Cards
▶ Books
▶ Board games
▶ Art supplies

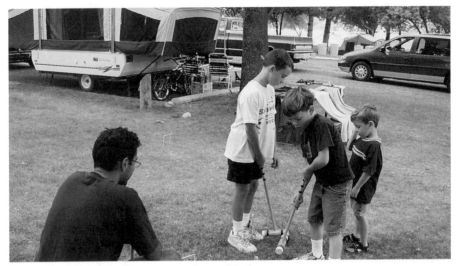

Bring a croquet set if your camp has a big lawn.

bats, badminton sets, Frisbees, tennis rackets, and horseshoes. Younger children bring their familiar sandbox toys, sturdy dump trucks, and tractors. Where there is water, you see inner tubes and inflatable boats. Bring some supplies for quiet times, too: books, art supplies, a tape or CD player with favorite tunes, a portable radio. Lots of people bring cards and board games.

While some parents take along lots of toys—Ellen allows each of her children to take one bag of familiar toys—others say that there is enough to amuse a child in camp without toys from home. If you know that you will be camping near a beach of some kind, digging and dumping toys are appropriate, unless you want your child digging and dumping with some of your eating utensils. Wendy advises against bringing new toys. When the whole experience is all new, there is comfort in old familiar toys. However, she warns, don't take toys that have lots of pieces, like Lego; stick to large, one-piece toys that are less likely to get lost, like Tonka road-building equipment.

Many small children, and older children, too, like good company best of all. Many families look for children the ages of their own kids to play with in camp. And many young people told me that what they liked best about camping was the opportunity to spend uninterrupted time with their families.

For more on what to bring for fun, consult the section What Should We Do for Fun? on page 170.

Miscellaneous Stuff You May or May Not Need

Trying to organize the long, long list of miscellaneous items that people take camping, I came up with a short list of categories. I have labeled these as items for safety, hygiene, comfort, first aid, or repairs.

Safety

Safety means finding your way around a dark campground at night as well as not getting lost in an unfamiliar park during the day. You should have at least one flashlight for each person. Some kids love having a flashlight of their own so much that it's not unusual for the batteries to run out in a single weekend. Be sure to bring extra batteries and extra flashlights.

A lantern, fueled by propane or white gas or running off of a battery, is good for the whole family. Gas and propane lanterns burn pressurized fuel in a mantle, a very delicate hood in which the fuel is consumed. If you're using this model, be sure to pack extra mantles; they are easily broken. The older models of these lanterns gave a very bright light, sometimes too bright, especially when it is coming from the campsite next door. Newer models are adjustable for brightness, but old or new, they should never be taken into a tent.

Battery lanterns have the advantages of being more portable. You can walk around carrying one without worrying about breaking the

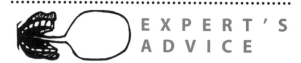

**E X P E R T ' S
A D V I C E**

Battery Operated

Some kids so love having a flashlight of their own that it's not unusual for the batteries to run out in a single weekend. Be sure to bring extras!

CHECKLIST
Miscellaneous Items

Hygiene

► Toothpaste and toothbrushes for all

► Soap and towels

► Clothesline

► Toilet paper

Comfort

► Pillows and stuffed animals

► Child carrier

► Lawn chairs and mats

► Heater

First-Aid Kit

► For details, see pages 88 and 204.

Safety

► Flashlights, batteries, and lanterns

► Whistles

► Walkie-talkies

Repairs

► Duct tape

► Sewing kit and lots of safety pins

► Miscellaneous pieces of tarp and lots of plastic bags

mantle, and you can take it into the tent. Some use rechargeable batteries.

A whistle is another safety device that many parents provide for their children. Don't put the whistles on strings around the children's necks; they could be strangled if the cord catches on a bush or a tree. Put the whistles on cords long enough to reach from their pockets to their mouths, pin the ends to the pockets, and stuff all inside.

You may see people on the trail and in camp with walkie-talkies. With their limited range, they're good for keeping track of the members of your party strung out along a hiking trail. But there are some problems with using them. If a hill gets in the way between two units, they can't reach each other. If the kids get hold of them, the batteries run down quickly. But if you're hiking in a flat area and you control the time on air, then walkie-talkies can be very useful.

If you're going to be hiking away from camp, carry some brightly colored trail-marking tape. Tie a piece to a low branch or a bush to mark the place where you turned off the trail or the fork that you took, so you can find your way back. Return trails look different than outbound trails. Look back often as you hike. On your return, untie the tape to use again.

Hygiene

In some families, toiletries are shared. One tube of toothpaste, one bar of soap, and one unbreakable bottle of shampoo is sufficient in an RV. Tent campers might want two of each, one for the boys' bathroom and one for the girls' bathroom, but everyone should have a toothbrush and a comb or hairbrush. (Although Sara, 11, told me that when she forgot her toothbrush, she shared one with her sister.) Other families pack a bathroom bag for each member, with all the variety of products that each person likes. All the bags should have a name or an identifying mark on them.

Wendy suggests that the bag that goes to the shower with you should have a hook so it can be hung up; if your bags don't have them, buy a small carabiner at an outdoor store and attach it to each bag. She also says that you should bring along extra waterproof bags so you can hang your clean clothes in the shower and they won't get wet. Campground shower stalls are not spacious and they don't have spacious dressing areas.

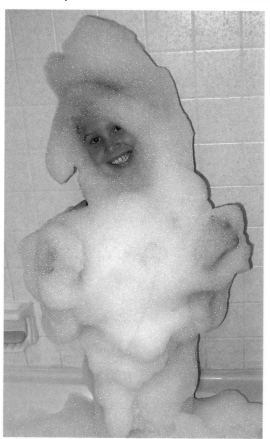

A camp bath can't be like this home bath.

Some campers bring along "sun showers," heavy plastic or vinyl water bags that sit out in the sun and absorb heat. Some models can be hung from a tree and come with hoses and shower heads for quick showers in camp. These would not work well in a camp with no privacy, unless you also had a sun-shower enclosure. All can be found in the Campmor catalogue.

Even if your washing product is biodegradable, you should not wash in a lake or stream, but dip some water into a basin, and when you are finished, dump it on bare ground. That means you'll need a basin, though some campers use one of their cooking pots for a wash basin.

Towels—lots of them if you will be swimming—are important. At Portland Luggage I saw a great big, rapid-drying micro-fiber towel that scrunches up into a tiny packet. It was dark blue, so it won't show the dirt. The whole family could share it.

A clothesline is handy for drying towels, swimsuits, and muddy clothes. Vicki's clothesline is a chain with a hook at either end; it wraps around the tree without harming it, and the hooks can fasten to any link, so it's adjustable. Some campers rig the clothesline as soon as they arrive at their campsite. Don't forget it when you leave.

Toilet paper is important, too; some parks provide it, some don't, and some run out. Bring your own to be safe.

Comfort

Everything that makes camping easier or cozier, that doesn't fit into any other category, could be called a comfort item—including pillows and stuffed animals, if these are important to someone in your family. Susan's family likes their pillows in the car. Ricki loves her big pillow. Backpackers often make a pillow by folding the clothing they remove in the stuff bag from their sleeping bag. Others carry inflatable pillows. Folding lawn chairs to be set up around the campfire or straw mats to roll out on the beach are comfort items, too.

> ### Quick Quiz
>
> #### Carrying Baby Comfortably
>
> **Q:** What makes a comfy baby carrier?
>
> **A:** Padded shoulder straps, a padded waist belt, and a storage pocket.

Candle lanterns give a lovely glow at the table, but they are no help when you're putting the tent up in the dark or walking to the bathroom at night. And candle lanterns should never be taken into a tent.

A gas heater is another accessory that never belongs in a tent. RV campers have the advantage here. RVs usually have heating systems. Some tent campers use battery- or generator-operated heaters in their tents, but I don't approve of that practice. Battery heaters

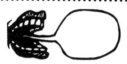

E X P E R T ' S   A D V I C E

Safe Lighting

If you bring a lantern for a "comfort" item, heed the advice in the Campmor catalogue: A burning appliance in a tent is dangerous. This includes stoves, lanterns, or heaters. Use only battery-operated lights inside a tent.

could still be dangerous in a crowded tent, and generators are noisy. If keeping warm is a concern of yours, take extra clothing, zip up the doors and windows of your tent, and let the person who feels cold sleep in the middle, between two warm bodies.

Finally, if you're camping with an infant, or perhaps even a lightweight toddler, you'll want some kind of carrier. You probably already own one for trips to the mall or the park. Is this a comfort item or a safety item? Either way, an infant needs a soft pack that fits on a parent's front; it should have some kind of support for the baby's head. As the child grows, if the head support is removable, you can face him or her forward in that same soft pack; soon that pack becomes too small, and you need to move on to a carrier for your back.

When you're looking at carriers, think about how you will get the child into it, how you will get into it yourself, and how comfortable it will be over a long period of time. If two parents are going to use the same baby carrier, it's important to make sure it's comfortable for both. Look for padded shoulder straps, a padded waist belt, and some kind of pocket to hold baby gear. You can often find a good-quality baby carrier at a garage sale, as other families out-grow their need for one.

First-Aid Kit

The first-aid kit is something that you hope you won't need, but you must have. (See more on first aid on page 204.) Maggie puts a bottle of water plus soap, a tweezers, antibiotic ointment, different sizes of Band-Aids, itch medicine, scissors, a nail clipper, and personal meds in a Ziploc bag.

I would add a headache remedy, a pain medicine like children's Tylenol, an anti-inflammatory dab-on cream such as hydrocortisone for insect bites, and something for diarrhea. You should also have something for blisters, either moleskin or one of the "second

C H E C K L I S T

What to Pack in the First-Aid Kit

▶ Soap and water

▶ Tweezers

▶ Antibiotic ointment

▶ Bandages in many sizes

▶ Scissors

▶ Nail clippers

▶ Moleskin or second skin

▶ Bug repellant

▶ Sunblock

▶ Your choice of products for headaches, pain, itches, insect bites, constipation, diarrhea, and dehydration

▶ All the daily personal medicines your family uses

skin" products. I also take a rehydrating product for excessive fluid loss through perspiration or excessive bowel action; in my kit, it's Gatorade.

If these products are not familiar to you, consult a pharmacist.

The pediatrician I consulted for this book added duct tape and a pair of latex surgical gloves. Duct tape fixes all sorts of things; the latex gloves are just as much to protect the first-aid provider as they are to keep wounds from being contaminated.

The first-aid kit is a good place for the bug repellent and the sun-block, two absolute necessities, and for the hand sanitizer to use after the outhouse and before cooking. Sarah and Henk Jr. agreed that mosquito repellent—the kind that you wear on your skin or your clothes—is indispensable. You need a different product to keep the bugs away from your picnic table.

If your children are prone to car sickness, try C-bands; those bracelets women wore for morning sickness are now available in children's sizes. Women should pack sanitary protection. Michael, who worked as a drug sundries representative, always had sanitary products in his glove box. Any time a woman in their camping group discovered that her menstrual period had arrived unexpect-edly, the word was always, "See Michael."

Repairs

Do you think you might need to make some repairs in the camp-ground? Bring a sewing kit, and put lots of safety pins in it for instant repair.

Jackie thinks duct tape is essential for camping. She once threw a roll into their gear at the last minute, and on that trip the zipper on their tent broke. It took them half an hour to get the tent flap closed with duct tape, which worked fine until someone had to pee. They unfastened the flap just enough so that person could crawl out and in, and they never again neglected to take duct tape camping.

While not exactly a repair item, there are many uses for plastic bags of all types and sizes. You can never have too many, and they take up very little room. You can use garbage bags or large grocery bags for packing clothes as well as groceries. Each meal that you assemble can be packed in its own bag, or you can have one large bag for breakfast foods, one for lunches, and one for dinners. More of them can be your trash containers in camp. Smaller plastic bags can hold condiments or art supplies. Take extra bags for carrying home the wet clothes and towels that didn't dry in camp. Ziploc bags will have all sorts of uses. You can cook in Ziploc bags, and the smaller size will hold treasures from the beach, as well as sandwiches.

Odd-sized pieces of plastic tarp are useful, too. You can spread them over the gear you leave outside at night to keep the dew off. Put a rock on top to keep it from blowing away. In a pinch, if you need a tarp and you don't have one, an opened garbage bag should work.

Packing

All of this gear requires containers. I made a special trip to talk to Wendy Liebreich of Portland Luggage Company in Portland, Oregon. Wendy gives workshops on packing for camping in RVs and in tents. She was gracious enough to spend several hours talking to me about how to pack, and I've added some of her ideas to those of my other experts.

RVs have built-in storage. Cupboards and drawers in the kitchen area hold all the essentials for cooking and serving meals. Ellen assigns one cupboard to each member of the family for clothing, and another one for toys and games. Some RVs have a closet with hanging space and towel bars in the bathrooms. Some have extra storage beneath the floor that open from the outside; Bridget calls this her "basement."

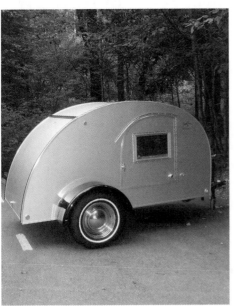

Families who own their own RV can leave their camping stuff in the vehicle all the time, ready to go. For those who rent an RV, however, Wendy suggests a soft-sided cloth bag for each member of the family. Wendy likes duffel bags, because they can be

This trailer doesn't allow for much storage. zipped closed and stuffed into odd-shaped spaces. She explained that assembling your stuff in one spot, emptying it into the RV cupboard, then collecting it all again to carry back to the house is a lot more work than just packing it in a duffel, putting the duffel in the cupboard, and then carrying the duffel back into the house.

Because things tend to get lost inside a big, dark duffel bag— Wendy called it "a large sea of emptiness"—Wendy suggests assembling similar goods in zippered plastic bags that have clear mesh

---

EXPERT'S ADVICE
Packing Tight

Expert campers often become expert packers. Follow Wendy's trick for reducing bulk: She uses compressor bags—plastic bags with a one-way valve—so something big, like a fleece jacket, can be squeezed to a flat package.

---

on one side. She puts her T-shirts in one bag, underwear in another, socks in a third. Clothing that is rolled and stuffed together won't wrinkle. Shoes should be in bags of their own, she said, down at the bottom of the duffel, where they would migrate anyway.

Wendy showed me some compressor bags, sturdy plastic bags with a one-way valve, so you can put something bulky, like a fleece jacket, in the bag, and then roll it to force the air out and squeeze it down to a flat package. These bags can be used over and over again. You can try the same thing with a large Ziploc bag by putting your finger in the "zipper" and pressing the air out, then quickly yanking your finger out and sealing the zipper. It's a little more difficult and you won't get as much air out, but it can be done.

RV owners who have smaller campers often complain that there's not enough storage room inside. Wendy recommends stuffing containers in any open space in the RV for traveling. Once you arrive in camp, remove these containers and store them under the RV. She also said many RV campers don't like to use the toilet or the shower in their vehicle if there are facilities in the campground that don't need to be cleaned (by them!). In that case, the shower stall and the toilet compartment can become additional storage areas.

Tent campers have to be more creative, although RV campers might use some of these ideas for their overflow or for their "basement" storage. Some families like the square plastic boxes with lids, some prefer canvas duffel bags, and others just use plastic or brown paper grocery bags. You also see laundry baskets, cardboard boxes, and suitcases. People use what they already have. I've seen campers use rubberized dry bags, the kind that rafters use, and open mesh bags. You can buy either of those in an outdoor store or from Campmor. At Portland Luggage, the mesh bags Wendy showed me had plastic over the mesh, so they would be waterproof. Vicki packs her gear in milk crates. When she arrives in camp, she empties the crates and turns them upside down to use as seats.

CHECKLIST

Packing Supplies

▶ Paper or plastic grocery bags

▶ Cardboard boxes

▶ Mesh or canvas bags

▶ Duffel bags

▶ Suitcases

▶ Lidded plastic boxes

▶ Laundry baskets

▶ Milk crates

There are advantages and disadvantages to each. Sara, 11, and her dad pack everything in Rubbermaid tubs with snap-on lids because these plastic boxes stack readily inside or outside. Another camper recommended stacking these tubs outside the tent where the contents would stay dry, but suggested that to keep the tubs really dry, you should cover them with a piece of tarp weighed down with a rock. However, these boxes take up a lot of room in the car. Laundry baskets and suitcases are also hard-sided and difficult to fit into limited spaces, and there is the expense of buying them.

Canvas or mesh bags, on the other hand, can be packed tightly together so you can fit more of them into your vehicle, and a full duffel bag can be a comfy backrest when you're lying around the fire. However, they will get wet from dew or ground water if you leave them outdoors overnight; they have to be stored in the tent or in or under the car.

Dry bags, unless you already own them, are expensive. Mesh bags are expensive too, but if you have them, you can see inside so you know where to find that T-shirt or sock that you're missing. Most of the other containers don't have that advantage. Plastic grocery bags will keep the contents dry, but you can't see into them when you're searching for something vital.

Paper grocery bags and cardboard boxes are cheap, compared to boxes or bags that you buy. The paper ones might melt in a rain storm; on the other hand, you can use the empties as fire starters or waste containers.

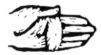

H E L P I N G   H A N D S
Personalized Packages

Your children can help with the packing by decorating or marking their own containers and by choosing the clothes and toys they want to take.

You can see into a milk crate, but if you want to use it as a seat, you have to empty all of its contents and leave them somewhere—probably on the floor of the tent.

Whatever you choose, it's wise to mark the container so you know what's inside. The kitchen box should be easily recognized among all the others. If you're traveling with a child still in diapers, be sure to pack a container for the used ones. (See the section on special concerns, page 98, for more about camping with an infant or a toddler.)

If each person has a box or bag, it should have his or her name on it, or a colored ribbon or some other personalizing mark. This is an area where the kids can help. Let them decorate their own container so they can find it later. The kids can also help pack their own things. If you want to limit the number of toys they can take, this is the time to do it.

This is also a time to teach the children how to plan for time away from home. Choosing what to take and helping to pack it will make the trip more exciting for the kids. If you're going to be gone for three days, they can count out three pairs of socks or three sets of underwear, with one more of each in case of an accident. Show them how you pack; are all your socks and underwear grouped together, or do you pack in layers, as some parents do, with one day's shirt, shorts, socks and underwear all stacked in a layer or rolled in a bundle together? Or do you put all the jackets, all the shoes, all the pajamas for everyone together in one bag?

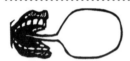

EXPERT'S ADVICE
Gear Care

Take advantage of sunlight to air and dry your sleeping bags and tents. Hang them outside if you can; if not, hang them in a dry open area.

Wendy suggests that children should have a complete outfit for each day packed separately in a zippered plastic bag with the child's name on it. Then at the end of the day, put the dirty clothes back in the same bag and put it back in the larger storage bag. All the child's clothes will be together, and the mud from today won't rub off on tomorrow's clean clothes.

All of these packed containers will take up lots of room. They are in addition to the tent, the rolled-up sleeping bags, and the hard goods like the stove and the folding chairs. You may need to add extra storage to your vehicle by piling stuff on the roof. Some people put their gear on the roof, cover it with a tarp, and tie it down with ropes or bungee cords. One of my experts told me a horror story of watching sleeping bags and other gear, not properly fastened, blow off the top of a car on the highway a few yards ahead of them.

A car-top carrier with a hard lid that fastens securely would be a better choice. Dobbie says that without their car-top carrier, they would never be able to carry all their gear in the family car. Before you start heaping anything on to the roof, check the owner's manual of your car to be sure you have the right fittings and that you don't exceed the weight limit for the roof. Check also that your car will still fit

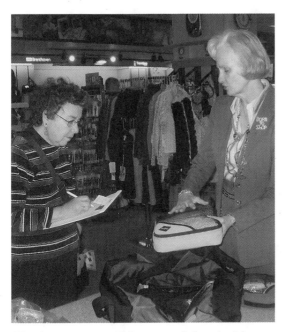

Wendy suggests packing a mesh bag inside a larger bag like a duffel.

through your garage door when the carrier is attached to the roof.

Be sure too that your car-top carrier is waterproof. Nan and Jack loaded their carrier with tent and sleeping bags, and set off to visit family in cities before their camping trip. They didn't pay attention to the summer showers that they drove through, because they were so sure their carrier was keeping the rain out. When they arrived in camp, around dinner time, they found their tent and sleeping bags were drenched.

Storage and Maintenance

Ideally, every family would have an airy place where tents and sleeping bags could be hung up out of season. Barring that, look for dry storage areas where your gear can be loosely stacked. Most tents come with a storage bag; before you pack your tent away for the week or for the season, make sure that it is completely dry and as clean as possible; don't ever put it away wet. Sweep or shake it out

C H E C K L I S T

The Indispensables

I asked all of my experts: "What is the most indispensable article that you take camping?" They came up with a wonderful list, a collection of items that you might never have thought of if you hadn't seen them here! You can devise your own list now, using my basics and their indispensables, eliminating the things that you think aren't important, and adding things that are.

▶ Maggie takes a roll of quarters for the shower, and a hammer for pounding in tent stakes.

▶ Ricki and Wendy take their glasses. Ordinarily, they wear contact lenses, but when they are camping, they can't manage proper eye care. They say it's easier to leave the lenses at home.

▶ Sara and her dad take small daypacks and water bottles, for hiking away from camp.

▶ Sisters Danielle and Elana bring books, lots of books. Some are for private reading, and some are for reading aloud. When the girls were younger, they took dolls when they camped, especially female action figures like She-ra, sister of He-man.

▶ Their mom, Sara, said her indispensable is bug block. Henk Jr. would agree with that. His indispensable is mosquito repellent, and he says many of his trips would have been unbearable if they had not been able to ward off armies of mosquitoes.

▶ My friend Goldie T. hangs sheets of Bounce brand fabric softener around the table to keep bees and wasps away. Zoe lights citronella candles. Madelaine also likes the soft, warm glow of candles, with some kind of wind screen so they won't blow out, but citronella has the added advantage of repelling insects.

▶ Marlene always camps in a site with an electric outlet. She brings her Christmas tree lights, and she and her kids make their campsite festive by stringing them up all around. She leaves them on all night, so they can find their way back if they go to the bathroom or walk the dog. She also brings an electric coffee maker.

▶ When Marlene's kids were smaller, she brought the kind of chair that clamps on to a table to create an instant high chair. Jeannie brought Christine's actual high chair; there was room for it in their tent camper.

▶ Some campers bring a mat or a piece of rug to lay as a door mat at the entrance to their tent, but Kate's dad has cut a large rug to fit the size of their tent; it makes the tent floor much warmer and more comfortable for sleeping.

▶ Vicki takes a baby yard—one of those folding devices meant to keep kids inside—and puts it around the campfire to keep kids back.

▶ Laura says a bell is necessary, especially if you're camping in bear country. When she walks to the outhouse at night, she rings her little bell as she goes, warning bears and any other critter to stay out of her way. (I have had a little bell attached to my backpack for years; I would never hike without it.)

▶ Backpacker Mike made the transition to family tent camping by buying, first, a bigger tent, and then a bigger car!

▶ Several RVers mentioned a broom and a dust pan. Sand and dirt on the floor can be a problem with kids everywhere, not only in an RV but in a tent, too. Some tenting parents instruct everyone to leave their shoes outside, under cover of course, to try to keep the tent clean.

▶ Betty's indispensables are the people. She has three grown children and five grandchildren, and they all really enjoy each other's company. They take one long camping weekend together each summer.

What becomes your indispensable? I'd really like to hear about it. Write to me in care of the publisher, Wilderness Press.

• •

to remove the debris that was tracked in. Hang it somewhere dry, like a garage or a basement, for a day or two. Better still, if the weather cooperates, hang it in the sunlight. Hang the tent as open as you can get it until it's totally dry.

If your tent needs washing, do that outdoors, too. Spread it out and scrub it with dish detergent and a sturdy brush, and rinse it with the hose. Hang it as you would if it were out in a rain; it may take longer to dry. After you wash it, you may need to reapply waterproofing.

Hang your sleeping bags, too, if you can; otherwise open them up to air in sunlight. Sleeping bags should not be stored tightly compacted in plastic bags; fold them loosely in breathable muslin bags, or simply roll them up on a shelf.

Many people never wash their sleeping bags! However, if you have children who wet theirs, you may have to. Sleeping bags are washable, but they require special handling. Down bags are especially fragile when wet; I take mine to a professional for washing. Bags made of artificial fibers can be washed, but they become very heavy when wet and might be too heavy for a home washing machine and dryer. My best advice is to take it to a commercial laundromat that has heavy-duty machines and follow the instructions on the tag on the bag. If you can't find a tag, call your local outdoor store and ask for advice about cleaning your sleeping bag.

Polyurethane waterproof material, often used for rain gear and for stuff bags, really begins to stink if it's tightly compressed. If you can't hang these items, at least store them loosely folded on a shelf.

One more precaution about tents: If your tent is old, if it's been in storage for some time, or if you bought it used, it may have leaky seams. Set it up outdoors on a dry day and squirt it gently with a garden hose from above, replicating a summer rain. Then check inside, and if there are leaks apply seam sealer where necessary. When it's raining in camp, it's too late to seal the seams or to put the rain fly over your tent.

While you're putting your gear away, make note of spots that need repairing, or better still, do it before you put your tent or sleeping bag away.

What About Our Special Concerns?

There are no excuses for not camping, although people try to come up with all sorts of justifications for not trying. Some say their children are too young, or that one member of the family is disabled, or that they follow a religion that has stringent requirements or that they can't leave their dog or that they are afraid to try this new activity all by themselves. But none of these excuses is valid.

I found, in my interviewing, many people who took their infants and toddlers camping, I found disabled people and religious people camping, and I saw lots of dogs in camp. I also talked to people who camped with friends, which is an ideal solution for hesitant, beginning campers. This section will cover those special concerns.

Camping with an Infant

No child is too young to take camping. An infant is probably the easiest of children to take. Randy and Tina began camping with their daughter when she was only three weeks old; she spent the nights in her car-seat carrier.

Many other babies have ridden contentedly in their safe infant carriers in the car, to continue in their hard-shell carriers or in comfortable front packs or backpacks worn by a warm, safe parent in camp. Infants are easily amused; a few favorite toys from home, a teething biscuit, a parent's voice, or just observing all the world around them keeps them occupied. Once again, this is a moment for imaginary camping. As you go through your infant's daily routine, mentally rehearse the same tasks in a camp setting. How will you bathe your child? How and where will you do diaper changing? Where will the child sleep? Where will he or she spend the days?

Packing for camping with an infant is little different than packing to visit grandma, except that you need to take fewer changes of fancy clothes. You do need sufficient changes, however, and you should allow for cooler temperatures at night. You also need the ointments or wipes or whatever else you use for diaper changes, and containers of hand sanitizer for the person who does the changing.

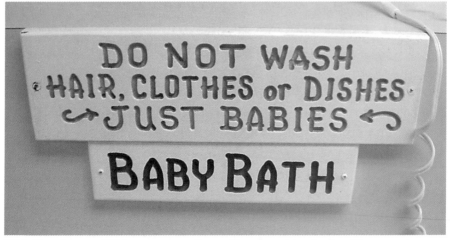

This Seattle-area KOA campground provides amenities for families camping with babies.

C H E C K L I S T

Camping with an Infant

Food

▶ Sufficient baby foods
  (cereals and jars)

▶ Feeding spoons and bowl

▶ Adequate supply of milk

Sleeping

▶ Car seat or play pen

▶ Blankets

Clothing

▶ Enough outfits, for both
  cool and warm days

▶ Sleepers or pajamas

▶ Diapers for the whole stay

Care and Comfort

▶ Small tub for bathing

▶ Play pen or ground cloth

▶ Toys

▶ Baby carrier

Diapers

Bring plenty of diapers, and lots of sturdy plastic bags for wrapping used diapers. The jury is out on cloth versus disposable diapers for camping, but whichever you choose, you will need some way of carrying them home or to the trash bins. Do *not* throw used disposable diapers down into the camp outhouse. Portable sanicans fill up quickly. If the privy is a hole in the ground, it takes forever, almost, for diapers to biodegrade, and every time the park service has to dig a new outhouse, it creates one more scar on the landscape. In fact, I believe that for short trips, all waste and garbage should be disposed of at home, to reduce the burden on under-supported campgrounds.

When I was writing *Backpacking with Babies and Small Children*, I did some research on cloth versus disposable diapers. I was pre-disposed to be anti-disposables, because they deplete forest resources. I learned that a lot depends on where you live. In Washington state, where we have lots of water and our used disposable diapers go into landfills, it makes more sense to wash and reuse cloth diapers. In a state like Arizona, where water is precious, it may be more environmentally sound to use disposables. If yours is a community where water is scarce and garbage is burned to create electricity, maybe disposables are a good idea. Unless we're willing to cart our babies around with no diaper at all, we try to make the best choice, the one that creates the least scarring and waste in the environment we live in.

Feeding

The food the infant eats in camp is the same as the menu at home. If your infant has been eating your mashed up table food, continue the practice in camp. Reconstituted dry cereals are popular foods for camping infants, as are bottled foods. Most parents discard unfinished foods because they don't trust the refrigeration of coolers, so you may need a few more jars than you would use at

IMAGINARY CAMPING

Camping with Baby

As you go through the daily tasks of caring for your infant, imagine doing the same thing in an RV or a campground. Think about simplifying those tasks. Does your infant really need a change of clothing several times a day? Would a gentle sponge bath work as well as total immersion?

home. Or you may feed your infant more of the jar, with less variety of foods at each meal.

Nursing mothers should be sure to keep themselves well-hydrated so that their supply of milk is not diminished. Even then, moms should be prepared to augment breast milk with formula, just in case the unfamiliar activities of camping lessen their lactation.

Parents of bottle-fed babies say they pack enough clean bottles for the trip, or they bring ready-to-use formula in a bottle, or they buy the kind of nurser that has a disposable plastic insert. Some parents boil water on their camp stoves and then cool it to mix with powdered formula, and some bring cooled boiled water from home. A few say that they actually wash bottles and nipples in hot water in camp.

Bottles may be a challenge, but washing the infant is easy in camp. Jeannie remembers bathing the infant Christine every evening in a small tub on the picnic table, with water heated on the camp stove. Some parks have a laundry room with a tub where parents have bathed their children. Other parents report that when the shower stall for the disabled in the park bathhouse had a seat, they carried their infant into the shower and bathed together. In the KOA campground that we visited near Seattle, there was an infant's bathing tub and table in the women's rest room. Parents who are camping in RVs would have none of these concerns. They could bathe their babies in the kitchen or bathroom sink.

All parents agreed that crawling infants could get dirty in camp. Some try to spread a rug or a tarp for the child, while Jeannie says she allowed her daughter to crawl on the dirt, knowing she would bathe her at bedtime. An empty, zipped-up tent with a few favorite toys inside is a fine place to keep a crawler while parents are busy in camp; most tents have a screen that can be closed while the heavier flaps are pulled back, so the child can see his or her parents. If you have room for it, a play pen is an ideal play space. A screen house is another possibility, but it means you're actually setting up two tents, one with solid walls, one with screens.

Sleeping

While Janetta had a play pen in her tent for her infant daughter to sleep in, many parents keep their baby in their own sleeping bags at night. When parents own zip-together bags, an infant can fit quite warmly and comfortably in the middle. Some families choose to sleep that way all the time, but babies who aren't used to so much togetherness sometimes want to stay awake all night and play, with mommy and daddy so close!

Be prepared for cold nights. A backpacker told me how they keep their baby warm at night by improvising a tiny sleeping bag from a down jacket: they pull the sleeves inside, lay the baby on top, and zip the front up to the neck; then they slip the wrapped-up baby into a stuff bag, put a warm hat on his head, and keep him between his parents all night long.

Closing the flaps on a tent or pop-up tent-trailer will keep the interior warmer at night. Parents who camp in RVs have an advantage: Their infants can be tucked into real beds, with a barrier of rolled clothing or towels to keep them from rolling off in the middle of the night. Some RVs have heaters, but if you use one, you must be certain that you provide adequate ventilation by cracking open a window or two.

Camping with Toddlers and Small Children

If infants are easiest, toddlers are the most difficult of children to camp with. They're not difficult in the sense that they won't enjoy the experience—but difficult because this age group requires the closest supervision. This is the age of discovery, but as the infant is content to merely observe, the toddler and small child will want to explore. For parents, the great pleasure of this age is seeing the world with fresh eyes; for the young child, everything is new.

• •

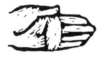

H E L P I N G   H A N D S
Official Duties

Allow children between the ages of 2 and 5 to help set up camp and participate in other jobs. Give them a title like "Official Assistant Tent Builder."

• •

Parents must constantly be alert. A child can admire a bumblebee, but not pick it up. He may be allowed to pick up a pretty stone but not put it in his mouth.

Children of this age are less content to ride in an automobile for long distances. Parents need to choose campgrounds fairly close to home, and allow for running-around stops along the way. Once they arrive in camp, children need to be occupied. Even though it may make the job take longer, they love to carry small items from the car to the table or tent site. They can "assist" the person putting up the tent by holding a pole or by handing him the hammer.

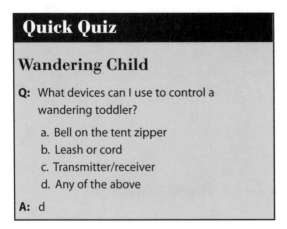

Quick Quiz

Wandering Child

Q: What devices can I use to control a wandering toddler?

   a. Bell on the tent zipper
   b. Leash or cord
   c. Transmitter/receiver
   d. Any of the above

A: d

The child who is in the midst of a potty-training regimen can continue that routine in camp, although accidents may be more frequent in the strange surroundings. Parents need to be prepared with extra clothing. Mike and his wife, camping with an almost-2- and almost-4-year-old, told me that the younger boy always wore diapers at night. His older brother sometimes stayed dry at night and sometimes didn't in "pull-ups." The boys didn't object to the outhouse, which had a metal fixture with a seat and a lid that looked something like the toilet at home. Some children don't like using outhouses that have unsavory smells, or the kind where the seat is a hole in a wooden box. To be safe, parents can bring from home a potty chair or at least the familiar small seat to set into the park's fixture.

Sleeping

Sleeping in the tent may be a scary experience for some children. My niece Beth, mother of three, told me of two experiences with children who couldn't fall asleep in a tent. When Sam was sleepless in his first year, they put him in his car seat and drove around the campground until he fell asleep. Then they carried him into the tent, still in the car seat, and he spent the night sleeping there.

Rachel was 2 when she wouldn't fall asleep in the tent, screaming and screaming. My niece sent Rachel's older sister to sleep with friends in the site next door. The following morning, at the water tap, an annoyed teenager said to her, "Did you hear that kid screaming last night? Must be terrible parents."

My niece replied, "That was my child, and I think I'm a very good parent."

The young man's mother, standing nearby, commented, "You don't remember what you were like when you were 2 years old."

Talking about the tent in advance and putting it up at home before your trip could avert a problem when night falls in camp. I know I'm repeating myself: Practicing with the tent is a wise idea on two counts—you need to know how to do it, and young children need to feel that it's a familiar space. If your tent is self-supporting, set it up in a family room or play room and let your young children spend time inside, even taking naps or spending a night there. Remember Vicki's memory of indoor camping, with her "campfire" made of crumpled red and yellow tissue paper, and a flashlight inside? You could do the same thing.

If your tent is outside, don't just set it up and take it down; leave it up for a while and let the kids spend time inside. Perhaps you can even spend a night, or part of a night, sleeping outside.

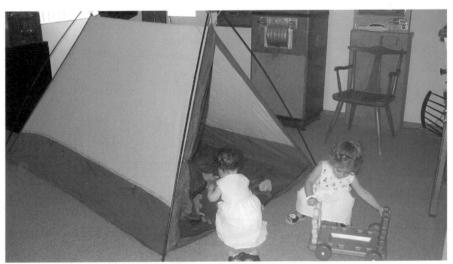

Practicing tenting at home helps make your tent a familiar space for the kids.

The strangeness of the tent may not be the problem if a child is afraid of the dark. Not only sleeping, but walking to the bathroom or even sitting around the campfire would be scary. At home, you may leave a night-light burning for this child; you can do the same in camp. Give the child a flashlight of his or her own, and allow the child to keep it on all night long. Bring plenty of extra batteries. If the light bothers other sleepers, arrange the bodies in the tent so that they see a minimum of light. If the light doesn't bother the others, you can even hang the flashlight from the highest point in the tent, so the entire "room" is illuminated. Do *not* try this with a candle lantern. Be sure it is a battery-operated flashlight.

While you may want to follow your usual routine in camp—meals at mealtime, naps at naptime—the newness of the situation may make your child unwilling or unable to wake up or go to sleep when you want her to. A quiet time, with a story, may suffice for a nap. Some parents take along a portable tape or CD player so their children can be soothed by familiar music.

Some children around the age of 3 are night wanderers; you'll know what I mean if you have one. They get up at night and walk around. If you have one of those, attach a small bell to the zipper of your tent so you can hear when anyone goes in or out.

If your wanderer is the kind of child who goes dashing off without you, the kind who runs away under the clothing racks at the department store, you may need a gadget to keep track of him. When my youngest was that age, I bought a little harness for him that had a leash attached. Though busybodies looked askance at us with comments such as, "He's not a dog," it was the only way I could take all three kids out in public by myself.

We tried a different kind of restraining device, a cord that attached to two bracelets, one on his wrist and one on mine, but he objected to that.

Now there is a better gadget, called Angel Alert. It's a small, battery–operated transmitter/receiver, with one for the parent and one attached to the child. The child's transmitter has a panic button, so he can radio a parent when he realizes he's gone too far. I saw it at

Portland Luggage; you can find out more about it through Travel Smart Angel Alert: 800-706-7064, www.angelalert.net, or www.franzus.com.

Camping with a Disabled Child or Parent

If families do their homework before the trip, camping with a disabled person can be just as much fun for all as it is for any able-bodied family. There are many kinds of disabilities; the person in a wheelchair will have different needs from the person with vision or hearing loss. There are many agencies, individuals, and a lot of information available to help plan a successful camping trip, but it may take some work to find them. Many of these resources are local, but you can go to national clearinghouses to locate them.

C H E C K L I S T

Campground Requirements for Disabled People

▶ ADA or family restrooms

▶ Raised tent platforms

▶ Paved paths

▶ Evening campfires or other activities the whole family can enjoy

Start with choosing the right campground. Use the internet or call or write to the campgrounds of your choice and ask them very specific questions. If you use www.reserveamerica.com to select a campground, you will find campsites marked with the international wheelchair symbol, and you should also find a telephone number that you can call for more detailed information.

The national Easter Seal Society supports 140 camping and recreational facilities across the country. Call 800-221-6827, or go to www.easterseals.org to locate your local society office. Ask them for information about accessible facilities in your area and talk to their experts about the camping needs of your family.

The website for the National Center on Physical Activity and Disability, www.ncpad.org, provides general information about camping for the disabled and can give you the names of agencies in your area that have programs or specialized equipment that you can borrow. On the website, go to Fun and Leisure: Camping, or call 800-900-8086.

Information on Camping for the Disabled

▶ National Easter Seal Society: 800-221-6827 or www.easterseals.com

▶ National Center on Physical Activity and Disability: 800-900-8086 or www.ncpad.org

▶ Disabled Sports USA: 301-217-0960 or www.dsusa.org

▶ For ADA-friendly RVs: Cruise America's "Fun Movers" (800-221-6827 or www.cruiseamerica.com) or El Monte RV (800-367-4808 or www.elmonte.com)

Disabled Sports USA is another clearinghouse for finding programs and equipment; their website, www.dsusa.org, lists organizations by state and indicates which ones have equipment available for use. You can also call them at 301-217-0960.

I found wonderful inspiration in *The New Mobility Magazine's Spinal Network: The Total Wheelchair Resource Book.* In a section called Sports and Recreation, there were heartening stories of wheelchair athletes. At the end of that section, there were six pages of resources for adaptive recreation and organizations across the country that provide all sorts of opportunities for the disabled. Although some of the activities may be geared toward adults, the information could be accommodated to kids. *Spinal Network* can be ordered from PO Box 8987, Malibu, California 90265, or look for it in your local library.

A Forest Service ranger in Washington state who has a disability himself told me, "Be articulate about your needs." Information is obtainable, but you may have to be persistent.

The Washington forest ranger told me that many of the existing facilities in his district are quite old . The Americans with Disabilities Act (ADA), passed by Congress in 1990, requires new construction or remodels to comply with ADA Accessibility Guidelines, but these guidelines are not very specific. Each agency interprets the guidelines for themselves, and then relies on their landscape architects to carry them out. In his district, a basic accessible campsite has a "hardened" surface—not necessarily paved, but not gravel or sand, either. It also has a table with an extended top at one end so a wheelchair could roll up to it. The toilets may be outhouses, but the door should be wide, there should be handrails inside, and there should be a ramp leading up to the door.

I visited two of the older Forest Service campgrounds in my area and talked to the professional hosts in each; they warned me that though some campsites had been set aside as accessible, they were still very rustic. Indeed, I found the outhouses to be not accessible at all.

All campgrounds are not the same. Surfing through the web, I found that accessible sites in Wisconsin state parks, for example, should be firm and level and have an accessible table, a cooking grill, and a campfire ring. The grill and campfire ring should be installed along the outside edge of the living area. At least one accessible campsite should be located near a barrier-free restroom and linked to it by a 5-foot-wide firm-surfaced path. An accessible drinking fountain and water supply should be nearby. The site should have electricity. Wide, level paths clear of debris would be important not only for the wheelchair-bound but also for those on crutches or those who are visually impaired.

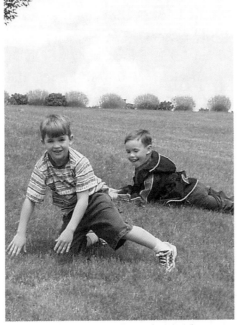

An accessible campground provides space for fun for the entire family.

In other jurisdictions, some parks had paved campsites and raised tent platforms so

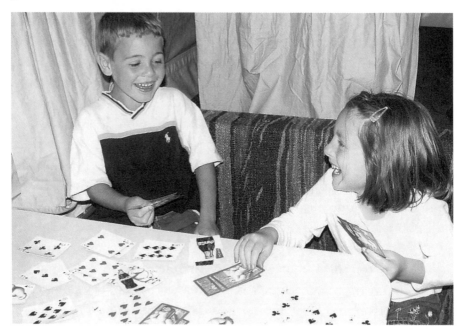

Playing cards is a great activity for camping families.

that a person in a wheelchair could transfer from the chair to the floor of the tent and crawl to a sleeping bag. Sleeping on the tent floor is not a wise idea for some disabled persons, so their families bring an air mattress or a cot for them.

If the family tent is a large one, a wheelchair can roll through the door to a camp cot; if the cot is high enough, the disabled person can transfer from chair to cot without assistance. Some families choose to camp in accessible yurts and cabins. Others rent the kind of RV where the back end folds down and a ramp slides out; although these RVs may have been designed for bringing along a motorcycle or an all-terrain vehicle, they work very well for rolling a wheelchair inside. Cruise America calls these RVs Fun Movers. You can find rental information for them at www.cruiseamerica.com or 800-671-8042.

If you're looking to rent an RV specifically designed to be wheelchair accessible, there are only a few agencies that I found that have such a rental. El Monte RV in California has two wheelchair-accessible units. These have electric lifts, special doors wide enough for a wheelchair to go through, and other hardware throughout the unit to make it usable by a disabled person. You reach them by calling 800-367-3687 or emailing traveltrade@elmonterv.com, or see their website at www.elmonterv.com. Their units can be picked up in California, Nevada, Florida, or New York. El Monte RV can install hand-control systems so a disabled parent can take children camping; they warn, however, that an able-bodied travel companion is required to operate some of the systems.

The less primitive the campground is, the more accessible it will be for the disabled. In Oregon's Jesse M. Honeyman State Park, which has showers and flush toilets, a notice on the door of the women's room declared that a person of opposite gender would be allowed inside if a disabled person needed assistance; that means a disabled woman could be helped by a man, or a disabled man could be helped by a woman.

At a Washington state park that I visited recently, the outhouse was also marked for accessibility; however, the concrete step up to the threshold was about 3 inches high, and I wondered whether a wheelchair user could get up without help. Because getting to a toilet is a major concern, many families bring their commode chairs along; if they have a large enough tent, they assign one of the rooms to be the bathroom. The Happy Seat Disposable Toilet (see Resources, page 242) would also be a useful product there.

I talked to Randee Young, the program director for SkiForAll, an organization in Washington that provides year-round adaptive outdoor recreation for children and adults with disabilities. Randee told me that their campers with vision or hearing impairments engage in all the activities of other campers. The techniques her organization uses for the physically disabled could be employed by any family with a disabled member.

When Randee takes groups camping, she looks for camps that have ADA or family restrooms, raised tent platforms, and paved paths. Where there are no platforms, they take big tents. She likes camps where there are evening campfires and other activities available. Her organization owns the largest fleet of adapted cycles in the Northwest, and she looks for long hiking trails for walking or cycling. These cycles are three- or four-wheeled vehicles for two, some side by side and some tandem, and they are available for families to rent. Her campers like water sports, canoeing, rafting, and fishing; special seating and straps make it possible for all to take part. Washington is fortunate to have an organization like SkiForAll; use your researching skills to find similar groups in your state.

Randee points out that parents already have lifting and transferring skills, so there's no reason why they should not take their disabled child camping. A disabled adult also should know his or her own limits, and within those limits be able to participate in family camping.

Camping with Other Families

Many of my experts report that camping with another family is the best way to go for everyone. Families can share their expertise on camping techniques; the children amuse each other so that their parents are excused from that task; and the parents, like the kids, have companions who are their own age.

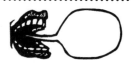

E X P E R T ' S   A D V I C E
Meals for Large Groups

Camping in large groups can make planning meals a challenge. Consider doing what Marlene's group does when camping: They always have a theme dinner, which could be bouillabaisse, pasta, or an ethnic theme, and everyone is responsible for contributing items or dishes for the group. To make the evening more festive, you might encourage people to bring appropriate table decorations or wear ethnic costumes.

When you have a number of families, everyone does not have to do the same thing all the time. If some of the group wants to play by the side of the lake while others go on a hike, the adults in the group can split the kids so all of them are supervised, not necessarily by their own parents. Some parents report that the kids actually behave better, with less complaining and whining, when they hike with somebody else's parents.

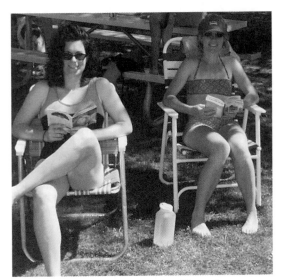
When camping with other families, the moms can take a day off while the kids are off with the dads.

Some families organize their time together around meals. Each family may be responsible for lunch or dinner on a given day, or, on a longer trip, each family takes responsibility for a certain number of breakfasts, lunches, and dinners. When Betty camps with her three grown children and their families, each family unit takes responsibility for a day's three meals—planning, preparing, and cleaning up. Grandma Betty's responsibility is to bring the snacks for the entire stay.

When Marlene's family camps, they also join several other camping families. On one night, they always have a theme dinner, where everyone brings something to share. When it was bouillabaisse night, everyone brought a different kind of seafood to add to the big pot. On pasta night, one person cooked a big pot of noodles, and the rest of the group had a pasta sauce competition. An ethnic theme brings a variety of Chinese, Mexican, Indian, or Thai dishes to the table.

Ricki and her family belong to a *chavurah*, a group of families who have been getting together for social, cultural, and religious events for many years. Those events have included camping together. They have had five, six, or seven families camping together, and once there were eight. Ricki was kind enough to invite me to meet with some of her group to talk about camping with other families.

Reservations are a must for this group because they want their multiple campsites close together. They don't try to leave the city all at the same time, but they arrive at the campground one after the other. Usually they camp Friday evening through Sunday. Early arrivals will pay for late comers so that they don't lose their reservations. (Ricki told me that one weekend their departures were delayed on a Friday afternoon, and they all ran into stressful weekend traffic. When they finally got to the park, no paired husband and wife was speaking to the other! They joked that they needed a marriage counselor to join their group.) There have been weekends, she said, when the last family arrived so late that the others stood around with flashlights, lighting their site while they put up their tent.

When their children were younger, the group camped about three times each summer. They were pretty casual about setting dates. One family would decide that they would like to visit a certain park, and they would send an e-mail to all the other members of the group. If the originating member wanted to reserve a group site, it was up to that person to reserve; otherwise, each family reserved a campsite for themselves, requesting a site near the others or doing it online where they could see a map of the camp loops.

During our meeting, which took place the day after Christmas, Ruth announced that she had a date and place in mind for next summer. She said she was going to reserve a group site as soon as the calendar allowed, and then she would let everyone know about it.

Ricki doesn't like group campsites because they often have outhouses instead of

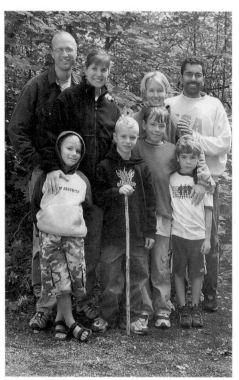

Camping with other families doubles the fun.

flush toilets, and the better bathhouses are far from the group site; she'd rather have everyone in the same campground loop. But other members said they prefer the group campsite because they are assured that they will all be together. Sometimes, they said, even though they all had consecutively numbered campsites, they weren't together, and sometimes other people were in with their group.

Ricki's group never shares meals. They say their kids have too many differing opinions to allow one family to choose a menu for all. It's just easier for each family to bring and cook their own

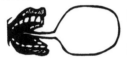

EXPERT'S ADVICE
Sharing Food

Even if you're not planning group meals, everyone in the group should prepare generous meals nonetheless. The children will wander from one family to another to see who is having the best dinner, and some people in the group inevitably forget some of their food. Besides, it's fun to see what other families consider camp food.

foods, except that the children tend to wander from one campsite to another to see who is having the best meals. They all prepare generous meals, knowing that the kids will come around and that some of families will inevitably forget some of their food. They all eat their meals at approximately the same time, and they do have a cocktail hour together before dinner, when everyone comes in from their day's activities and they share hors d'oeuvres.

The people who met with me all had their favorite memories of trips they had shared. Some of them remembered camping near lakes, when they brought inflatable rafts, inner tubes, and life vests. Others recalled a hike that turned out to be longer than expected; they switched children to reduce the complaining, although one person commented that his child was "an equal-opportunity whiner" who would hike and complain with anyone.

When the children were smaller, the parents entertained them with storytelling and singing. Sometimes the children would put on a show with little skits. They put the kids to bed early and they would wake up with the sun.

Now that their children are older, the kids stay up late playing cards, and when the sun comes up, they sleep in. Now the children bring friends whose parents aren't part of the group, and the group camps less often. They are more likely to go to a lodge or rent a houseboat together. (See Beyond Camping, page 223.) Some in the group are concerned about too much togetherness among their teenage children. Formerly, it was not unusual for the kids to leave their parents' tent and share smaller tents. Now these parents don't want a boy and girl off in a tent by themselves!

I asked the group if there had been any problems over the years. They said that at times when a family had not shown up in camp they didn't know whether to assume that the family wasn't coming or to pay their reservation fee to hold the site. Now that they all have cell phones, that isn't a problem.

Then I asked the group how they had all managed to remain friends and spend time together over many years. They said it was important to camp with like-minded people. Although they joked about the idiosyncrasies of some members who weren't present (the woman with the huge first-aid kit, the man who boiled water every morning to wash his hair), they were pretty tolerant and accepting of each other. They said their main reason for camping was to be together; when there was more than one family, it was more fun just hanging out.

Bringing the Dog Along

You will see lots of dogs in campgrounds. Having the dog along may be trouble, but this furry family member earns his place in the tent by making the kids in the family so much happier in strange surroundings.

It's just as important for your dog to ride safely to camp as it is for the other members of the family. Norman's dog always rides in his carrier in their motorhome. Most dogs aren't trained to wear seat belts or other restraints. Will your dog sit quietly on the rear seat of your car or in the RV? If not, consider putting him in his car carrier for the trip. Like the kids, the dog needs opportunities to get out and run around in the course of a long trip; don't lock him in the car while you go off.

Your dog may be well-trained, but he doesn't understand camp rules. It's up to his owners to make sure, first of all, that dogs are allowed in the park. Some beaches do not allow dogs. Some parks where migrating birds rest do not allow dogs. Ask whether some areas are off limits to dogs. At the same time, there may be areas where dogs are allowed to run free. At a KOA campground I visited, there was a fenced off-leash lawn for dogs.

Pick up your dog's poop in a plastic bag and drop it in the garbage can. Don't allow your dog to chase chipmunks or squirrels or other wild animals, and keep him quiet, especially at night. There's a lot to bark at in a campground; your dog may be excited by all the strange smells and sounds. It's up to you to keep him calm.

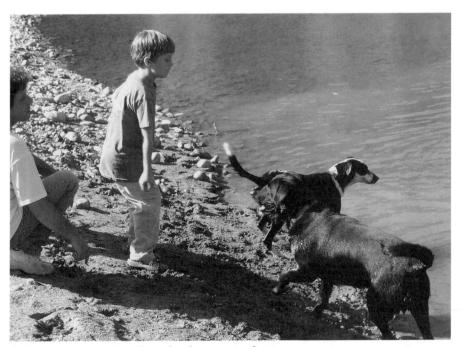

Kids may be happier when the dogs come along.

Keep your dog from annoying other people, especially children. Most parks require dogs to be on a leash at all times. He may be a wonderful, friendly animal, but if the child in the campsite next to yours is afraid of dogs, your pet bounding over there isn't going to help him overcome his fears. Bonnie has trained her dogs to walk

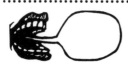

EXPERT'S ADVICE
Fido-Friendly Travel

If your dog isn't trained to sit on a seat wearing a seat belt, put him in his carrier for the trip to camp. When you stop to allow the kids to use up some of their pent-up energy, let the dog run, too.

behind her, rather than in front. When she gives the command, "Trail dogs," they know to drop back, even when they are on a leash.

You can ignore those rules, of course. Owners tell me, "She hates her leash," or "We live in an apartment; he never gets to run free." That's nice for the dog, I suppose; the dog doesn't know about rules. But think about this: What kind of example are you setting for your children? If you want them to grow up thinking that laws can be observed selectively, and that you don't have to obey the laws that aren't convenient for you, don't be surprised if your kids grow up to ignore your rules or the laws of your community.

Religious Observance

It's not unusual to see a family sitting around the table at their campsite, hands joined in prayer before a meal. Many families continue their daily religious rituals when they are camping.

My friend Habib, a Muslim, told me that he carries a prayer rug wherever he goes. Five times a day, he finds water to wash, spreads his blanket facing toward Mecca, and prays. If he can't find water, he can cleanse himself by rubbing with sand. On a camping trip, he uses his compass to find the right direction for prayer. Sometimes his children join him, and sometimes they don't.

Jews observe dietary laws by keeping meat and milk products totally separate; they observe their Sabbath from sundown Friday night until sundown on Saturday by refraining from lighting fires or lamps. Susan's family is able to follow these rules by eating only dairy meals while they are camping, and by organizing their trips for Sunday through Tuesday. Sara's family packs two separate coolers, one each for meat and dairy; they let their campfire burn down on Friday night and they don't use flashlights until Saturday evening. Sarah told me that she often takes her coffee pot to a neighboring campsite on Saturday morning and explains why she can't heat her coffee on her own stove. No one has ever refused her use of their stove or campfire.

On Friday evenings, to mark the beginning of the Sabbath, Jews light candles. Vicki told me this story: A Jewish family lit their candles, but no lantern or flashlights. The other families camped around them, noticing their darkened campsite with two candles burning on the table, came rushing over, saying, "Did you forget your lantern or your flashlights? We have extras you can use."

I've included this story because, while a few campers have tales of raucous, ill-mannered neighbors, most campers share the same values of love for the peace and quiet of nature, and they are out in the woods for quality family time. If you have questions about how to camp once you arrive at your campsite, you will probably find the other campers willing and eager to assist and teach the novice or inexperienced camper.

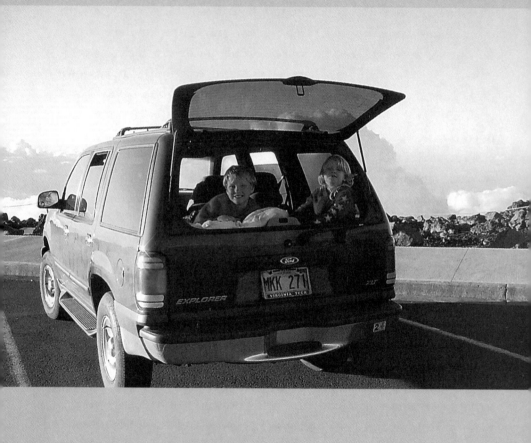

The Real Thing

- ▶ Are We There Yet?
  (Safe and Happy on the Road)

- ▶ How Do We Set Up Camp?

- ▶ What's Life in Camp Really Like?

- ▶ How Do We Cook in Camp?

- ▶ What Should We Do for Fun?

After weeks or possibly months of planning and imaginary camping, you're finally ready to set out on the real adventure. This section pulls together all the plans and ideas you have been storing up. We begin with the road trip, and then go on to set up your camp, enjoy the campground, and take your camp down. This section will give you all the nitty-gritty details of life in camp, with an emphasis on preparing meals and having fun.

Are We There Yet?
(Safe and Happy on the Road)

The first day of a camping trip goes something like this: pack the car, drive to camp, unpack the car, settle in. Don't plan to do a whole lot more than that, but try to make the whole day fun for the kids. The fun should begin on the way, with games in the car that involve the whole family, and, if the trip is a long one, opportunities to get out of the car and stretch or run around.

Packing the Car

My friend Max used to be very particular about how he loaded their van for vacations. He was so particular that one year the family set out a whole day late, because Max had packed and unpacked the van so many times!

You don't have to be like Max. You should have a good idea about what goes where before you begin to pack for your trip.

Sometimes it's easier to get big jobs done without "help" from the kids, but even small children want to pitch in when it's something as exciting as packing to go camping. Besides, packing is part of preparing your kids for the trip. If you have small children, let them bring a few items out and pack them in the RV or the car. They can carry boxes of cereal or bags of marshmallows to the RV kitchen; they can carry the toys they chose for the trip out to the car. In the evening, put the kids to bed early and finish packing

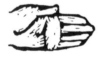 **H E L P I N G   H A N D S**
Packing Tricks

Let the children carry a few items out to the vehicle you are packing. Finish the last of the packing while they're sleeping, so everyone is ready to go in the morning.

while they are asleep. When they wake up next morning, you'll be all ready to go.

A safety note: Make sure your RV or your car is parked somewhere safe for children. Don't park your RV on the street if the entry is in the rear; back the vehicle into your driveway so that the

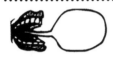

E X P E R T ' S   A D V I C E

Do You Have All the Pieces?

Double check your tent to be sure you have packed poles and stakes. Sandy and Pat arrived at their campsite and discovered that they had left their tent poles at home. They were able to rig a kind of lean-to, but it wasn't as windproof or cozy as a tent.

children won't step into the street going in and out. Same thing for the car; if the children will be bringing things to the trunk or the rear doors, park the car in the driveway or garage where they can reach the rear without stepping into the street.

If you have an RV, the packing is much easier. The kitchen things go in the kitchen cupboards. The clothes and toys go into each person's assigned spaces. The big toys—bicycles, trikes, fishing gear—go into outside compartments. Sleeping bags can be stowed on top of the beds, jackets hung up in the closet. Juice goes into the refrigerator and snacks are handy in the kitchen. Everything you need is easily accessible.

When you're traveling in a car, you have a more difficult planning task. Some things need to be available in the car for immediate access. That may be juice in a cooler, snacks that don't need refrigeration but need to be close, and possibly milk and a diaper bag with all the usual changing accessories for an infant. You may want to have a few toys or books for the trip, and also jackets or sweaters in case you run into cool weather. Susan's family likes to have their pillows in the car.

Are you planning to have a picnic lunch on the way to the campground? Don't bury it under a pile of sleeping bags!

At the same time, think about what you will need when you first arrive at your campsite. Those things should go into your car last. That means packing your tent in a place where you can retrieve it first thing when unloading your vehicle. If it's raining or threatening rain when you arrive in camp, you will want the tent and perhaps the dining fly to be up before you remove anything else from the car. You don't want all your bedding, kitchen boxes, clothing duffels, and anything else that's in the way sitting out in the rain while you struggle to get the tent out and up. As a last precaution, check your tent to be sure you have the poles and a sufficient number of stakes before you put it in the car.

••

Five Things to Do
While Traveling in a Car

1. Singing

2. Listening

3. Number games

4. Alphabet games

5. Geography games

••

Are you planning to arrive in camp at dinner time? When family members are tired and grouchy from sitting in the car for a long time, they're going to want to eat right away. This may not be a good night for cooking over a campfire. Many of my experts bring a quick dinner for the first night out—cold chicken, fresh vegetables cut and packed at home, and fruit and cookies for dessert. After their camp is set up, they take the time to build a small fire and make s'mores.

Fun on the Way

Some teens and pre-teens are occupied and isolated in the car or RV with individual CD players, videos, and electronic games. They can amuse themselves for hours at a time with these gadgets. However, a good number of parents, especially those with very young children, want their kids to be involved with the family and aware of the scenery. The people I talked to had a lot of good ideas about how to keep kids happy while traveling, using their ears, their eyes, and their quick minds.

Music is a good way to hold children's attention. The whole family can sing along with favorite tapes or CDs, or they can sing the old songs that their parents sang when they were young. Teenagers may sneer at these, but younger children still love to sing with their parents such songs as "Old Macdonald Had a Farm" or "I've Been Working on the Railroad," or "She'll Be Coming Round the Mountain," especially when there are appropriate snorting or hooting sound effects. Ambitious parents can create a guessing game, "Name That Tune," by recording bits of well-known songs on a tape or CD, and playing it in the car.

Reading aloud is a more quiet diversion on the road. I remember a trip from Seattle to southern California, where I held three children, ages 2, 7, and 9, and their father spellbound with the story of *Hitty: Her First Hundred Years,* by Rachel Field. When I visit that 7-year-old, now an independent woman living in another state, I still find that wonderful book on her shelf. Not everyone can read aloud in a moving vehicle, so suitable stories on tape or CD that everyone listens to also work well.

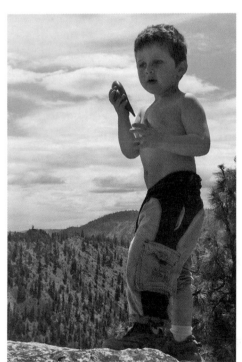

Looking out the window provides a wealth of material for in-car games. "I Spy With My Little Eye" is the easiest. Take turns spotting something along the side of the road. "I spy something red" may be a stop sign or a barn. "I spy something brown with legs" could be a horse or a cow. It's important to give as many easy clues as possible so that the youngest player will feel like a winner.

Be sure to stop along the way to let everyone stretch their legs.

Many people told me about counting games, which are good for short or long drives. In the simplest version, the children choose something—the American flag, blue cars, horses—and together count each one they see. The next step is to allow each child to choose something different to count; younger children may just call

....

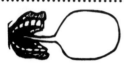

E X P E R T ' S   A D V I C E

Twenty Questions, Eighty Miles

On the road? Try my favorite road game, "Twenty Questions," or one of its many variations, such as "Animal, Vegetable, Mineral." These fun games will make the miles fly by!

....

out, "I see a cow!" or, "I see a barn!" but to make the game a little bit competitive, the one who sees the most of his or her chosen object wins a prize—a box of raisins or a bag of M&Ms.

Another version of this game is "Prediction," where an older child, 7 or 8, tries to predict the number of these objects he will see before you start out. The one who comes the closest wins the prize. On a trip that covers many days, each child can count the numbers of a certain kind of car—Volkswagen beetles, convertibles, pick-up trucks—or of a specific fast-food restaurant—Subway or Dairy Queen—and keep track of their daily totals; the winner is determined at the end of the journey.

Alphabet or number games can be communal or competitive, according to the wishes of the family. In these games, the children are on the lookout for something that starts with each letter in the alphabet in order—an apple tree, a barn, a cow. Older children can be working on their own, with the first child who calls out the apple tree allowed to go on to B, while the others have to find a different apple tree or an appliance store sign before they can go on.

In the number version, everyone looks for a commercial sign or a license plate that has numbers. With younger children, the whole family might work their way through the series: "I see a 1." "I see a 2."

Janetta and her daughter played a license plate game in which they tried to make words from the letters on the plate. On a recent long trip, my car load were entertained by noting the names emblazoned on the fronts of all the approaching RVs and campers: Monarch, Westwind, Sleep Queen. We made a game of it: Look at the next two RVs you see. Who would you rather travel with, a Diplomat or a Buccaneer?

"Going to Grandma's" is a variation of the alphabet game, and it's also a memory challenge. The person who starts says, "I'm going to Grandma's and I'm going to take an apple," or something else that starts with A. The next person says, "I'm going to Grandma's and I'm going to take an apple and a beanbag." As you go through the alphabet, the game gets harder and harder. This can be a competitive game, with the person who misses dropping out, but on a long trip it is probably a better idea to keep everyone in the game by giving little memory hints. When the game is over, if you get that far, you can do a challenging reverse alphabet: "I went to Grandma's and I left my zebra, but I kept the yurt and the x-ray and the window..."

"Geography or Place Names" is another game for older children who have studied some geography. The person who starts calls out a geographic name, like Washington. The next person has to find a name that starts with the last letter in the previous name: Nebraska. Then it gets tough, because a lot of the geographic names that start with A, also end in A—Alaska, Alabama, Albania—and someone really smart has to think of Akron. This game can become competitive, with the last person who can't think of a place name losing, or it can be a communal effort, with everyone working together.

The old favorite "Animal, Vegetable, Mineral" is a variation of "Twenty Questions," which is another good car game. In "Twenty Questions," the questioners have 20 chances to guess what the leader is thinking of. In the "Animal, Vegetable, Mineral" variation, the questioners might spend their first two questions asking, "Is it an animal?" No? "Is it a vegetable?" No? Don't waste your third question—it must be a mineral. Then you go on to ask, "Is it in this car?" "Is it in our house?" An added value to the game is that children learn what constitutes animal, vegetable, or mineral.

You can also create your own games. Ellen, who is a graphic designer, creates beautiful cards to entertain and challenge her children on long trips. Every day, each child selects one card from a brightly colored envelope. "Did You Know?" cards give information about the area they are visiting or about some of the famous people who have lived there. Ellen's "Destination Challenge" cards develop map and math skills: They list the day's destination and ask, "Which roads should we take? How far is it? How long will it take to get there? Where do you want to stop for lunch?" These cards also challenge the children's imagination: "There is a park in Arizona called Dead Horse Ranch State Park. How do you think it got its name?" Another card asks, "Was Butch Cassidy a criminal or a folk hero?" And the cards always end with, "Let's talk about it!"

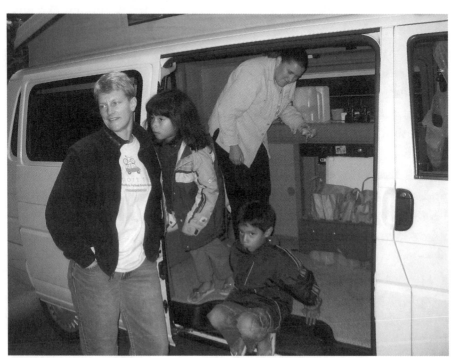

Arriving at camp provides a welcome end to the drive.

Ellen's cards are bright and attractive, but you don't have to be a graphic designer to create similar questions for your family; the tourist information packets you ordered from the state should give you all the facts you need.

Ellen also has developed a series of scavenger hunt games called "Seekers" that other parents could emulate. Ellen's games are designed for Seattle and for San Juan Islands, in Puget Sound, and one more will come out soon for Maui. Her game cards show pictures of sights, large and small, in a given neighborhood; players earn points by locating the objects and answering the question on the back of the card. You can learn more about these games at her website, www.famboomerang.com.

Whatever game or games you choose, try to avoid the kind that involve giving a tap or a rap to another participant. In the *Seattle Times*, I read an article on games in the car that suggested "Slug Bug." Whoever is first to spot a VW Beetle gets to administer "a sharp rap" on the arm of the non-spotters. I can imagine the chaos that would have created among my kids if we had ever allowed them to do that!

How Do We Set Up Camp?

At this point, you may be asking that age-old question: Are we there yet? Yes, finally, we are there! We have arrived at our campground. We check in at the gate to find our reserved campsite and pay our fee. If there is no gate, we drive around the loops, looking for the site with our name on it, knowing that the ranger or host will come around to collect if we don't find him first. If we didn't make a

The First Four Things to Do at Your Campsite

1. Set up your tent or level your RV.
2. Orient your family to the campground.
3. Set up your kitchen.
4. Set up the dining fly, shade, or screenhouse.

reservation, there is a challenge. We drive around the loops looking for the best campsite, the one that will please everyone, taking into account all the variables like where the bathroom is, how far it is from the lake or the beach, how much shade there is, how much sun, how much privacy from the campers next door.

The kids may want to explore the park before they do anything else, but most of my experts agreed that setting up your own personal home away from home, the tent or the RV, must come first. After that, you can explore, take your time setting up the kitchen, and make your "home" more comfortable.

Setting Up in a Tent

There are two bits of advice about tents that I have been stressing throughout this book: First, the best preparation for camping in a tent is just that—preparation! You should have become so thoroughly familiar with your tent before you ever set out on your camping trip that it goes up in no time. You should have practiced putting it up more than once in your yard or in a park, so you can do it in a hurry in a rainstorm and in the light of your headlamps at night. This practice is an activity the whole family can do together. That way, young children grow familiar with their temporary home while you learn how it works.

Second bit of advice: Pack your tent last, so you can pull it out of the car first and set it up.

So, having followed my advice, when you arrive, you are ready to go. There is a lot of "work" that the kids can do, especially putting up the tent, even though the job may take a lot longer with their help. If there is no designated tent pad, kids can help choose where the tent

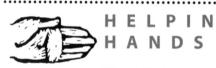

HELPING HANDS

Tent Setup

Here are four things your child can do to help pitch the tent:

1. Clear the ground.
2. Spread the ground cloth.
3. Hold a pole.
4. Pound in a stake.

CHECKLIST

The Perfect Tent Site

▶ Is it level?

▶ Is it private?

▶ Is it out of the wind?

▶ Will the terrain protect it from pooling water if it rains?

▶ Will putting our tent here damage the environment?

should go. Even if there is a tent pad, you don't have to pitch your tent there if you don't like it. Michael and Ricki said that their spacious three-room "condo" tent is often too big for the tent pad. Diana and Larry once put up their tent on the space intended for the car, which was more level than the tent pad. If your tent is self-supporting, you may set it up in the middle of your site, and then pick it up and move it around, trying out different spots.

This is an opportunity for kids to learn some basic camping concepts, like finding the most level ground. My kids used to lay down on the ground to see if they would roll. If you can't find a perfectly level spot, if there is such a place, put your tent where your feet will point down any slope.

Here are some other questions to ask your kids when you choose a place for your tent: How private is this spot? Can passersby see into it? What will the prevailing wind do to our tent? You don't want the wind blowing directly into the tent door. Ava, 11, remembers the "never tiring wind" making the sides of her tent flap in her face all night long. Maddy, 12, remembers moving their tent behind a bush in the middle of the night so the wind wouldn't blow it over.

Look around the tent site for signs of water flowing. Is the site in the route of water running down from a higher place? If the site is low and level, it may become a big puddle when it rains. Does it have many trees around it? If you think the night might turn cold, you're better off pitching your tent under some trees, where the cold night air and dew won't descend on you. If it's going to be a hot night, you might want your tent in the open air.

Finally, is the chosen spot on bare ground, or is it on grass or foliage? Plants in campgrounds take a real beating over the camping season. Teach your children to protect the living ground cover in camp by not walking on it and certainly not pitching a tent there.

There are many tasks children can do to help set up the tent. They can inspect the tent site and remove any pinecones, rocks, twigs, or other irritants that might poke up during the night. Kids are good at that. To help preserve the floor of the tent and make it more comfortable, lay a ground cloth down and set the tent up over it. Kids can hold a pole while a parent pulls the guy rope out and stakes it. If the tent has poles that are threaded through pockets, kids can help push the poles. Kids can hold a stake in place while a parent pounds it into the ground; or a child can start the process of pounding the stake, and a parent can finish the job.

After years of having his young son "help" pitch the tent, Michael realized that his son now knew how to set it up all by himself. "I looked over at him, and I realized that we were working together," he said. "It was wonderful."

As soon as you put up the tent, cover it with the rain fly, even if the sky is clear. The rain fly should stretch beyond the edges of the ground cover. Otherwise, rain falling on the ground cover will run into the tent. If the ground cover is too wide, tuck it up around or under the edges of the tent. Do not dig a trench around the tent; years ago that was the custom, but today it is considered a destructive practice.

Once the tent is up, you can decide who will sleep where and spread your insulation and sleeping bags in assigned spaces. Children adapt more readily to sleeping on the ground than their parents do, as long as they have some kind of insulation—a foam pad or thick newspapers—to keep the cold and damp away. Parents may require an air mattress to soften the ground, or, if the tent is large enough, even a cot. Some mattresses come with pumps that can be attached to the car battery, so the task of blowing up the mattress is much easier, but blowing up an air mattress, at least for the first few puffs, is a task that many children enjoy.

It is impossible, I truly believe, to keep a tent floor clean inside. Nevertheless, some people try to do this by laying a piece of carpet or floor mat just outside the tent door and leaving all their shoes outside.

If you brought a dining fly for your picnic table or a shade gazebo, this may be the time to set it up, or you may wish to wait until more urgent camp tasks are finished. My family always waited to do this unless we thought rain was imminent. The dining fly is tricky to set up; at least two corners must be tied to trees. Depending on your campsite, the other two corners can be tied to trees or anchored to the ground. It's not a fun job to do when people are hurried or hungry or both.

Setting Up in an RV

If you arrived in an RV, you must park it in the designated spot at your campsite and level it. If your RV isn't level, your appliances won't function properly. You should have learned, before you got this far, how to work the jacks that level the RV. If you get in trouble, ask the other RV campers around you for help. They will be

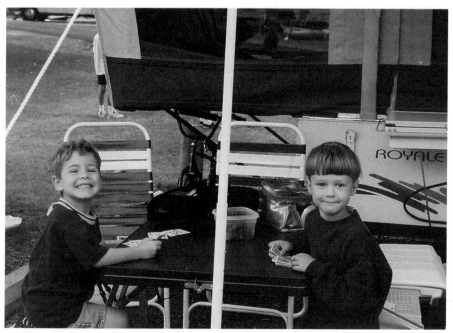

RVs have built-in space for extras like a table for a game of cards.

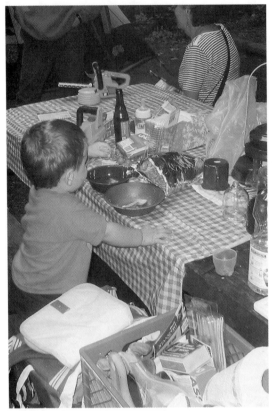

One of the most important things to set up early is the kitchen.

happy to assist you; people who belong to RV organizations, like the Good Sam Club, take pride in their ability to help new RV users.

When that task is done, connect the RV to the water, power, and sewer lines and switch your appliances to the new power source. Next, pull out your side awning, and, if you brought a table to use under it, set it up now.

If your campsite does not include a full hookup, you need to carefully monitor the use of the resources you have. If you're in a dry camp, without any resources at all, you need to watch the level of water you're using. If there is an outside source for water, you may want to carry water to your RV for washing, and save the water from home for drinking and cooking. Unless you have a generator for electricity, you also need to keep an eye on your battery discharge.

If you have electricity and water but no sewer, you need to keep track of the use of your toilet and waste water, so that you don't overload your holding tank. When Vicki's family rented an RV, they were told that the toilet's tank would hold 50 flushes and then they would have to dump. They posted a sheet of paper in the toilet compartment where everyone was supposed to mark each time they flushed. Whenever anyone stepped out of the door, the others would ask, "Did you mark down the flush?"

Campground Orientation

Once you know you will have a roof, either cloth or solid, over your head when night comes, you have a little more leeway in your first day's activities. At this point, you can take a walk around the campground—a little tour of your space. Are there bathrooms or outhouses? Where is the one nearest to your campsite? Is there a water tap? Where is it? Does it have a drain next to it where you can dump your dishwater? Find the water supply and, while you are there, fill a water container to take back to your kitchen. Find the garbage cans and take a good look at them; in many campgrounds they are designed in clever ways to keep animals out.

C H E C K L I S T

Campground Orientation

Find the following:

▶ Nearest bathroom or outhouse

▶ Nearest water supply

▶ Nearest dishwater dump

▶ Nearest garbage cans

This is the time to set up your family rules and boundaries. How far from your campsite will you allow your children to wander? If you allow the kids to go beyond your own campsite, show them how far they can go. Walk the boundaries with them and explain how far they may go by themselves. If you expect them to stay within your own campsite, make that very clear. Some parents mark the boundaries by scratching a line in the dirt or by tying up plastic tape (which they take down when they leave), pointing out the tree or the hedge that marks their borders.

In some parks, I have seen gangs of children on bicycles and tricycles riding freely through the campground loops. At what age should your children be allowed that privilege? You must decide, based on your judgment of your child's judgment and his or her riding ability. You could bring your own bicycle and ride the loops with your kids, or you can walk alongside the tricycle rider. I saw one family who had harnessed their big dog to pull a tricycle, while Dad held a leash.

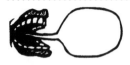

EXPERT'S ADVICE

Keeping Food Away from Critters

Backpackers often store their food by hanging it from a tree to keep it out of animals' reach. You probably won't have to use this technique in a drive-in campground, but hanging the food is one job that children love to help with. To hang your food from a tree, you need a sturdy bag, a long rope, a rock, and an old sock. The kids can try throwing the rock over the branch, and then help pull the bag up.

First, you have to find the right tree with a perfect branch. You want your food bag to hang at least 12 feet up from the ground and 10 feet out from the trunk of the tree. Put a rock into an old sock and tie it to the end of a long rope. Throw the rock over the perfect branch that you found and let it fall to the ground. Make a contest of throwing the rock up; you may be surprised when your teenagers are suddenly able to do it.

Next, place the food in a sturdy bag—a sleeping bag's stuff sack works well. If you're worried about keeping the bag clean, line it with a plastic garbage bag. Remove the sock with the rock and tie the rope to the food bag. Together, you and your children can pull the free end of the rope to hoist the bag up to the branch. Finally, fasten your end of the rope around the tree.

Setting Up Your Kitchen

Is all that exercise making you hungry? Before or after your orientation walk, you should set up your camp kitchen. RV campers will be finished with their lunch before the tent campers even get started, because the RV kitchen is already set.

In some families, the kitchen-parent quietly sets up the kitchen while the tent-parent and the kids are noisily setting up the tent. But if that didn't happen, the whole family can work on getting the kitchen workable. This is a part of the camping trip where even the smallest child can be involved; be sure to acknowledge the help that all hands deliver when they cart that box of cereal or bag of marshmallows from the car to the picnic table.

Unless you are stopping at an extremely primitive site, there should be a picnic table for your use. Park tables are usually built with attached benches down each side, but not across the ends. That's to keep people from walking off with the benches, but it makes working at the tables difficult. You can set up your kitchen any way you like, but walking through a lot of campgrounds, I've noticed that most people use one end of the table as their work area, the middle for storage, and the other end for sitting and eating. They set up on the benches as well as on the tabletops; nobody sits at the kitchen end.

The camp stove should be at the working end, with pans and utensil nearby. Foods that need cooking are stored close to the stove, but foods such as fresh fruit can be down at the sitting end. The table is often covered with plastic tablecloths and there are covers over the foods that are out.

The water container sits on one edge of a bench, so that any water that spills or drips will fall on the ground and not on the table. (At one campsite I visited, two little boys were happily filling dump trucks with mud that was created by a drippy water jug.) Some campers set out a bucket to collect wastewater, and dump it properly all at once.

Five Vital Posts in a Camp Kitchen

1. Stove
2. Water supply
3. Food
4. Garbage container
5. Wastewater container

Make a plan for disposing your wastewater. We're talking gray water here—water that was used for washing dishes or vegetables or people—*not* toilet waste. Toilet waste, from potty chairs or dirty diapers, should be carried to the bathroom or outhouse. (However, you must not dispose of the diaper in the outhouse, just its contents.)

Dishwater, which contains not only soap but also fats and food particles, should be dumped in a drain near the water spigot. If there is no drain near the water spigot where you are camping and there are no signs telling you where to dump wastewater, pick a discreet spot at the side of your campsite where you can dump. Try to strain the food particles out of the water first and throw that waste in a trash can. If left on the ground, those food particles may attract unwanted critters to your camp.

Don't even think about dumping wastewater in the bathroom or the outhouse. Some camps have a sign in the bathroom saying that people should not dump wastewater there. Roz says she likes to choose a plant that looks as if it needs water, and pours her water out there. Never dump your wastewater into a lake or a stream. Even if you are using biodegradable soap, you should dump it in a drain or on the ground.

You should also set out a garbage container, possibly just a large plastic bag. Let the children know that their discarded candy or cookie wrappers should go into the bag and not on the ground.

Your first meal in camp may be lunch or dinner, but when you are finished, don't just walk away. Dirty dishes, food, and garbage are all the same to the wild creatures that share your campground. Before you do anything else, store your uneaten food in your cooler or in the

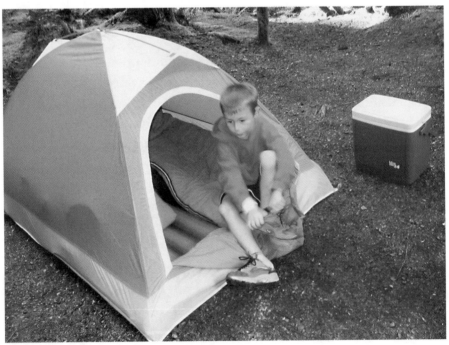

Keep your tent clean by leaving shoes outside.

food container. Wash your dishes and discard the dishwater properly. Carry your garbage to the garbage cans. If you're going to leave the campsite or go to bed, put your food somewhere where an animal can't get to it. Ricki saw a flock of crows attacking a picnic table where the campers had gone off and left their meal out. If your campground supplies animal-proof storage, put your food there. If not, lock it in your car or put it in a bag and hang it from a tree.

Making Your Campsite Comfortable

Once the basics are taken care of—setting up your RV or tent and establishing your kitchen—you may want to make your campsite more comfortable. A lot depends on how long you plan to stay; if it's just for one night, you may not want to bother. But after you have put up your tent, eaten and cleared away your first meal, and everyone has had a walk through the campground, it's a good time to set up the dining fly or shade canopy over your picnic table.

If you brought a dining fly, use rope to attach each corner of the fly to something solid, like a tree. If you plan to set it up as a lean-to, fasten the lower two corners down, either by staking them, tying them to a bush, or weighing them down with a rock.

Shade canopies and screen houses are self-supporting, but they need to be staked down so they don't blow away. If your picnic table sits on a concrete pad, so that you can't stake the canopy down over it, weight the corners with rocks or small bags filled with dirt or sand.

A much easier way to make your campsite comfortable is to bring out the folding chairs, light a small campfire, sit back and enjoy the evening.

What's Life in Camp Really Like?

For kids, everything is an adventure when you're doing it out-doors and alongside a parent. As Randy, a dad, told me, "Mundane tasks become exciting." Everything they do in camp should also be a learning experience for your kids. Randy involves his 6-year-old daughter in every task. When they set up the campfire together, he is teaching her about fire building and fire safety. She rolls up the paper fire starter, helps gather little twigs for kindling, and even starts the flame with a long-handled barbecue clicker.

This section covers the everyday life in camp and how you can teach the kids to manage daily tasks from morning until night, from keeping clean to going to the bathroom outdoors to napping to good manners in camp. We'll help you break up your camp at the end of your stay, and then reflect on establishing your family's camping traditions.

Quick Quiz

Napping without Sleeping

Q: What's almost as refreshing as taking a nap?

A: Spending a quiet break in the midst of an exciting time.

Days in Camp

On your first day in camp, setting up the tent, unloading the car, carrying items to the picnic table or to the tent site, setting up the kitchen, and inspecting the campground may be all you can do. Make those tasks fun. All the camp chores that seem like drudgery to the parent who has done them many times are new and exciting to the child who has never done them before. Bringing water to the campsite may be work for a parent, but a child who helps filter the water from the stream, or who has a hand on the handle when the bucket is carried back from the tap, is having a different kind of experience. Collecting little twigs for the fire is another job that kids and parents can share. Young Sarah likes blowing up her air mattress. For her five kids, Stephanie said, the business of camping is what it's all about.

On your second day in camp, you're ready to start your first full day's camping adventure. You know the kids will be warm later in the day, but when they wake up they may say they are freezing. Dress them in layers of clothing that can be removed as the day wears on. If the kids will be wearing shorts and a T-shirt in the middle of the day, put that on them first. Put a warm sweatshirt and sweatpants

over the shorts, and a warm jacket and hat over all. That should keep
them warm through breakfast. As the sun comes out and the day
grows warmer, the layers peel off. By lunch time they may be down to
the T-shirt and shorts. Whatever you do during the day, take a ruck-
sack along so someone can carry the discarded clothing.

Decide how and where you are going to spend the day. Take
advantage of your park's locality. If you're camping in a forest, take
a hike. If you're at the seashore or at a lake, go down to the beach.
If you're in a historic area, visit the ruins or the house or the vista
and talk to your kids about what happened there and why it is sig-

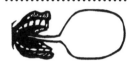

EXPERT'S ADVICE
Making Camp Chores Fun

Camp chores that are routine to parents are new and exciting to children who have
never done them before. Involve your kids in everything from setting up camp to
making dinner by creating manageable tasks for them to complete. There are many
learning opportunities in camp, and doing daily tasks outside is a completely new
activity for kids.

nificant. If you think you're going to be gone for the whole day,
pack a lunch to take along. Even if you plan to return to your campsite for lunch, take along some drinks and a few snacks. The section
on fun activities, page 170, will give you many specific ideas for
what to do with your children.

Time moves more slowly when you're camping. The children's
schedules are much more simple: no school, no daycare, no running off to ball practice or music lessons. Some events, however,
continue, like three meals a day, naps, and bedtimes. You and your
children will decide how rigidly you want to follow your usual day.
Mealtimes will be roughly the same: Breakfast certainly will be
shortly after waking up. Lunch can be a sit-down meal at your
campsite, or you may do what Susan's family does. They sleep in,
eat a substantial late breakfast, and then snack through the rest of
the day until dinner.

Naps may or may not happen. Children who usually nap can lie down on a mat in a tent or in the RV, but that's not to say they will sleep. An RV can be darkened and cooled. A tent sitting in the sun becomes very warm inside, not conducive to napping. A screen house would be a comfortable place for an infant to sleep, but it may be too bright for a toddler. If your child slept in the tent at home when you were practicing with it, he or she is more likely to take a real nap in camp. If you have a tape or CD player, you can bring some familiar quiet songs to listen to and, with luck, your child will fall asleep. However, even if he or she doesn't actually sleep, the quiet time will be refreshing in the midst of an exciting new experience.

Keeping Clean

Ordinary hygiene is different when you're camping. Your standards may be looser, but some tasks, like brushing teeth, should not be abandoned.

When a campground has a bathroom, it's not unusual to see people walking down the road in the morning with a towel over an arm and a toothbrush in hand. It is possible to wash and brush your teeth in a public bathroom, but many campers prefer to take care of those tasks more discreetly, at the back of their campsite.

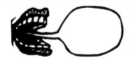

E X P E R T ' S   A D V I C E

Keen and Clean

Don't count on always finding soap, hot water, towels, or toilet paper in camp bathrooms. Bring your own supply or bring hand sanitizer to use in lieu of soap and water.

In some families, the first adult awake in the morning fills a teakettle and puts it on the stove to heat. It doesn't take much warm water in a wash basin with soap and a washcloth to clean up enough for a day in camp. You sometimes see men shaving in front of a mirror hung on a tree. When the washing is done, you can brush your teeth and spit your toothpaste into the wash-water

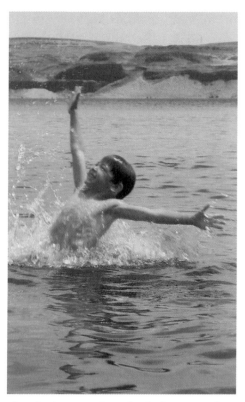

A swim is not quite a bath, but more fun.

container, to be disposed of properly. Campers tell me that one basin serves a lot of functions. They wash themselves, the dishes, and the baby all in the same basin.

Here's another way to have your kids brush their teeth outdoors: Teach them to use their heel or a stick to scrape a little hole in the ground in a bare place where no plants are growing; as they brush, they can spit their toothpaste into the hole and then cover it up and stamp on it. Children like the novelty of spitting into a hole, and they are much more cooperative about brushing when they can do it that way.

Some families take care of their kids' major daily cleaning in the evening, because it's too cold to wash in the morning. Mornings are cold in many campgrounds, especially those in the mountains or on the shore. The kids crawl out of their warm sleeping bags to straggle down the road to the bathroom or the outhouse, and return for just a quick wash. That teakettle on the camp stove provides warm water for a breakfast drink when they come back as well as for the morning wash-up.

Ricki said that when they are camping for just the weekend, nobody is too concerned about staying clean. If the campground has coin-operated showers, they take their handful of quarters and shower. Otherwise, they wait until they get home. Michael said they aren't intimate when they're camping, so it doesn't matter if he doesn't smell good.

A coin-operated shower will give you so many minutes for each quarter. Read the directions carefully, and pay attention to the timer. With some meters, the first quarter gives you less time than subsequent coins, so if you run out of time before you're finished, it costs more to start over again. Worse still is to run out of quarters when you're still soapy. If you're washing your hair, or one of the kids is in the shower with you and you're washing her hair, you need to plan for plenty of time to get all the shampoo out. It might be a better idea to do the hair washing at your campsite. Heat some water on your camp stove and use the all-purpose basin for a more relaxing shampoo. Or wait until you get home.

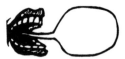

E X P E R T ' S   A D V I C E

Keeping Downstream Clean

Here's something to think about: We all live downstream. Help keep lakes and stream water clean by washing up and disposing of soapy water far from natural water sources.

Campers in an RV have no excuses for not staying clean. They have a bathroom sink where they can wash and brush their teeth, and they have a shower. RV shower stalls may be narrow, and sometimes they share a compartment with the toilet, but the water is warm and if they're connected to a water supply, campers can have a relatively generous shower. Just remember to remove the toilet paper roll from the stall before you begin your shower.

Deborah told me how to shower in a dry camp, where the RV is not attached to a water supply and you have to use water from your tank. "You do it fast!" she said. First, you wet yourself all over, in about 30 seconds. Turn off the water, and soap yourself all over. Turn on the water again for just one minute and rinse off most of the soap. If you don't get it all off, Deborah said, that's all right, you can wipe it off with your towel.

A dirty face is not a big problem in camp. Dirty hands are not a problem either, most of the time, but after using the toilet and just before eating, it's a good idea to have clean hands. Some park bathrooms have running water, hot and cold, and also soap and paper towels or hot-air dryers, but don't count on always finding them. Some parks have only cold water; with budget cuts, many no longer provide soap or towels. When the kids return from the bathroom or the outhouse, it's a wise idea to be prepared with warm water and soap in the basin, or else carry a big supply of some kind of hand wipes or hand sanitizer.

Whatever you do, do not wash in the lake or in a stream—even if you are using biodegradable soap. Dip some water up in a basin, wash in the basin, and then dispose of the water properly. At an outdoors conference, I saw a booth set up by an organization that lobbied for clean water. Their slogan is, "We all live downstream." Think about it. Explain to your children that the water in the little stream or lake in camp will run down to bigger streams and lakes until it becomes the source of drinking water for cities and towns far away.

Toileting

As you move out of your campsite for your day's activity, carry toilet paper, wipes or hand sanitizer, and a plastic bag for used toilet paper wherever you go. If there are no indoor toilet facilities at your destination, teach your children how to relieve themselves in the woods.

Tell them to choose an area of soft ground that is at least 200 feet (100 big steps) from any stream or lake, and dig a hole 4 to 8 inches

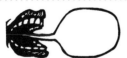 **E X P E R T ' S   A D V I C E**
How to Poop and Pee in the Woods

1. Walk 100 big steps (or more) away from any lake or stream.

2. Dig a little hole to poop in and cover it when you are through.

3. Carry your toilet paper out.

4. Pee on bare ground.

deep there. Some people carry a little trowel for digging the hole, but you can also do it by kicking your heel into soft ground. Tell them to squat over the hole so that their poop drops into the hole. When they are done, they should fill the hole with the dirt they removed and stomp down hard. Have them drop their used toilet paper into a plastic bag, and clean their hands with a wipe or sanitizer. Drop the wipe into the bag with the toilet paper.

Some children, especially those who are newly toilet trained, have a difficult time relaxing enough to defecate over a hole in the ground. Some parents carry a little toilet seat that they put on the ground over the hole; this "bear's potty" is more familiar and easier to use than bare ground. (I didn't intend that pun!) Other parents have built up rocks and logs to create a little throne that a child can sit on.

In any case, it may be difficult for the child to poop, even though she has a strong feeling that she needs to go. Parents need to be patient in a situation like this, sitting with the child, talking quietly while you wait for action. If there are older siblings around, impatient to move on, it's best to let one adult go on with the older children while another adult waits with the needy child.

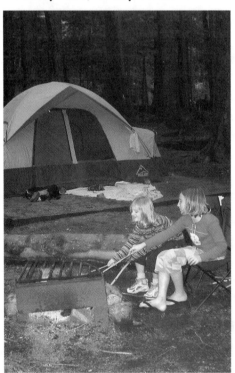

A campfire is the perfect place for social hour.

Urine is less polluting than fecal material. In fact, the urine of a healthy person is sterile, but it's still not acceptable to pee in a lake or stream. Teach your children to find some bare ground and pee there. Little girls should drop their toilet paper in the plastic bag. Most people would prefer to step off the trail to urinate, but in Olympic National Park, the rangers advise visitors to pee right on the trail. They say that the goats and deer in the park love salt, and when urine evaporates on plants, an animal will chew the plant to the ground in order to get the salt. The soil on the trail is already barren, so urine there soaks into the ground and no plants are destroyed.

Evenings in Camp

Evenings in camp are, for many parents, the best time. Dinner has been eaten and cleared away. There is a warming fire going in the fire pit, and the adults are sprawled in comfortable folding chairs. The kids are riding their bikes safely around the camp loops, because there is hardly any traffic at this hour, or else they're playing quietly at your campsite. The Italians have a saying for this, *dolce far niente*, the sweetness of doing nothing.

You can try to put the kids to bed at their usual bedtimes, but more likely the children will go to bed later than usual and their parents will go to bed earlier. When everyone is sleeping in the same tent, it can be disturbing to have someone come in late, so parents need to set everything up so they can find their night clothes and crawl into their sleeping bags as quietly as possible. Keep your shoes handy; you may be walking someone to a toilet in the middle of the night.

RV campers have it easier: The kids go to bed in their own spaces, their parents have more room to stay up late in their space, and the walk to the toilet doesn't require a trip outdoors.

Bedtime routine is the opposite of morning. The kids are cleaned up a little bit. They brush their teeth and visit the bathroom or outhouse. They dress or are dressed in appropriate sleeping clothes, and they're tucked into their sleeping bags. Young kids get a song or a story. Everyone gets a flashlight to keep close at hand in case they awaken in the middle of the night.

Each night, parents clear the campsite. They check to see that all the foods and garbage are put away where animals can't get them.

They douse the fire and make sure that anything that could blow away, like a table cloth or a towel, is firmly weighted down, even if there is no wind at the time. Folding chairs should be folded and put under the table or the RV, and the awning on the RV should be rolled up. It's better to do these tasks now when it's quiet rather than at 2 a.m. when a gale-force wind is blowing.

Michael likes to put everything portable, like the cooler and the lantern, out of sight in the car or under the table to discourage thieves. Nothing has ever been taken from his campsite, but he doesn't want to tempt anyone. Ricki puts her glasses in her shoes, where she can find both easily if one of the kids needs to be taken to the bathroom in the middle of the night. My tent has a pocket in the side seam where my glasses spend the night. At last, the parents, too, crawl into their sleeping bags for the night.

Good Manners in Camp

It's important for your children to learn good behavior and consideration for others in camp. Children are never too young to start learning this.

Some parks give more privacy than others, with a hedge or a bank of trees between campsites, but sometimes you will find yourself living very close to your neighbors, with no visual barrier in between. Teach your children not to run through other people's campsites and not to stare into them. That's easy enough to say, but when some people pitch their tents right next to the trail to the beach or the bathroom, it's hard to walk past without noting the supplies left on their picnic tables or their laundry on the line. Try to be as unobtrusive as possible when you must pass close to others. If the trail leads to the bathroom, teach your children to be as quiet as they can be when using the

Four Problems Among Neighbors in Camp

1. Noise
2. Bright lights
3. Lack of privacy
4. Speeding

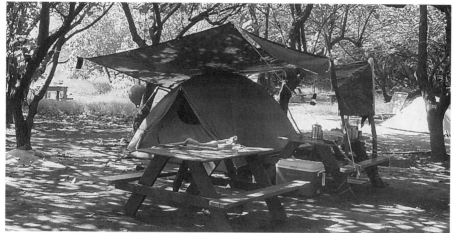

The campers at this site can relax quietly under their shade fly.

trail at night. Tell them to shine their flashlights only on the trail, and not into other people's campsites.

In many state, national, and private parks there are rules about noise, bright lights, and speeding through camp, and there are rangers who enforce those rules. But in other parks, it's up to the campers to apply their own rules of good behavior.

Noise can be a problem when people are living close together. We may tell our children to use indoor voices when they are indoors, but here they are not indoors. Shouting may be acceptable, outdoors and during daylight, but after the sun goes down, voices should go down, too. The people who like to stay up late singing around their campfire should remember that they may be preventing the early risers next door from falling asleep.

Campers in RVs who have stereos and television sets should turn the volume down, and campers who put their radios or stereos on the picnic table should turn them down or even off after 10 p.m. People who string up Christmas lights around their campsite—not exactly a wilderness experience—should be aware that campers around them might find them intrusive. The lights are less annoying than the whine of the generators that might be running them. Many camps have rules about turning generators off between 10 p.m. and 6 or 7 a.m.. Even a lantern that gives off very bright light may illuminate the campsites on either side of your spot, to the annoyance of your neighbors.

So after you have taught your children not to run through other people's campsites and to keep their voices down at night and to avoid shining their flashlights into other people's campsites, what is suitable behavior when your neighbors don't have the same sense of propriety that your kids have?

A respondent, who shall be nameless, told me that she put her child to bed in the tent at nightfall, but the bright light from next door sent weird shadows on the walls that frightened the child. She asked the neighbors to turn off their lantern, but they refused. However, they did move the lantern so less light crossed over into her campsite.

The same respondent told me of another incident, where she asked a group of young men camping next to her if they would move their noisy evening gathering to a different campsite (they were spread out over several). One of the men, she said, grew very upset at this and deliberately banged pots together and slammed the lid on their cooler and otherwise made lots of unnecessary noise, but they did move to a fire pit down the road.

I can't help wondering if this woman was perhaps a little too demanding of the people around her, and I wonder how her requests were couched. It isn't easy to confront strangers about their behavior, especially when everyone is looking for an enjoyable experience and we all have different ideas of what makes a good time. Conflicts can be avoided sometimes by choosing your campsite carefully. If you're settled with your young children and you see a group of young adults moving in next door, you might try to ask them, politely, to find a different campsite. Conversely, if you and your small children move in next door to a party of young adults, you might ask them for quiet after 10 p.m., but you can't really demand an earlier quiet time.

Speeding through camp is a different matter. Privacy, noise, and bright lights are issues of comfort. Speeding is potentially dangerous.

When there are small children playing in the roads, don't ask, tell the speeders to take their activities elsewhere.

Going Home

When you're ready to leave your campsite, the process is the reverse of starting out. Everything that you brought needs to be re-packed, either in the container it arrived in, or in a family laundry bag or garbage bag. The children can help in gathering up their goods, but if they lose interest, keep some of their toys out until the last minute. If you're in a hurry or if it's threatening to rain, keep them occupied coloring or playing a game at the picnic table while you pack the car.

Once again, the tent goes in last. Try to clean it out a little before you pack it, by sweeping it if you have a broom, or by shaking it out if you can manage to lift it.

C H E C K L I S T

Five Things to Do Before Going Home

▶ Pack the car or RV.

▶ Douse the campfire.

▶ Dispose of garbage and wastewater.

▶ Inspect the campsite.

▶ Stop at the bathroom.

Put out the campfire. Spread the coals in the fire pit, and sprinkle them with water. Stir the coals and sprinkle again. The fire should be so cold that you can put your bare hand into it. Remove any garbage in the ashes. There shouldn't be any, because you should not burn garbage, but if you see a foil wrapper or something else that didn't burn, pick it out and put it in the garbage bag.

Dump your wastewater in the proper place; if it's soapy and not dishwater, you can dump it on the fire, but dishwater with floating bits of garbage needs to go into the drain. Check to see that your clothesline is down and packed; it's an item frequently forgotten.

The last thing to do before you take off is a camp inspection. The whole family should take part in this exercise; it is a learning experience in taking care of our heritage. Is your campsite in just as good, or better, condition now than it was when you arrived? Walk around the campsite looking for things left behind; "things" can be as small as a candy wrapper or a twist tie. Look for telltale signs that you were there. Is there toothpaste on the ground? Cover it. Is one of the kid's collections lined up neatly? Scatter the pieces.

Take your garbage to the garbage can or pack it to dispose of it at home. Make sure your fire is completely out. Make one last stop at the bathroom. Then have a safe trip home!

Family Traditions

After you return from your first camping trip, you're ready to plan for the second. Ask your kids what they would like to do the next time you go camping. Don't be surprised if they want to repeat something they did the first time. Repeat it once, repeat it twice, and suddenly it becomes a family camping tradition.

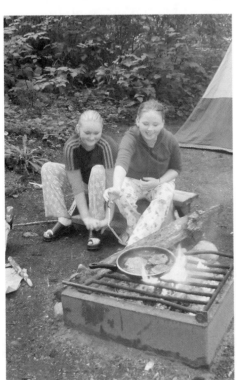

Grilling your meals can be a great camp tradition.

My family's camping traditions revolved around places and food. We returned many, many times to Jesse M. Honeyman State Park on the Oregon coast. We always stopped for lunch at the same pancake house on the way there, and more recently we have made a point of visiting the aquarium in Newport, Oregon, too.

A student told me her father wakes up early, gets a big fire going, and serves hot cocoa to everyone as soon as they wake up.

Sara's family has a tradition of reading aloud. Danielle and Elana told me that their dad is a wonderful reader who does lots of different voices. They love to sit around the fire in the evening, listening to him read.

Michael tells stories, about Green Goo the Vindow Viper and Murphy the Wonder Dog. His children and the other children in their group of camping friends love to hear his stories over and over. In their group, one couple is famous for their pancakes. She makes very thin crepes, filled with canned cherries, while he makes "fat pancakes." The group expects both kinds when they camp together.

Your family's traditions will be different. Maybe it will be Dad fixing chocolate chip pancakes. Maybe it will be Dad cooking, period! Don't be surprised if what your children remember is something that appeared to be very minor at the time.

How Do We Cook in Camp?

Cooking outdoors. Cooking and eating outdoors. Cooking and eating outdoors not on a patio or deck. That seems to be the magic of meals in camp for children. The same kids who might balk at chores in the kitchen at home love to participate in meal preparation outdoors in camp. Almost all of the sixth and seventh graders from the classes I visited commented in their essays on their memories of cooking their favorite foods in camp, and their parents remember how the kids were willing to help there.

Camp Stoves and Fire Pits

Susan and Bill cook all of their meals on a wood fire. They bring dry wood from home or buy it in camp. I asked Susan what she would do if the camp didn't sell wood, and she said most campgrounds are close to a store and her husband would drive back to get it. Susan doesn't use the grill that is sometimes in place in fire pits. Her husband is adept at building a fire that burns down to a flattened surface, and Susan places a big cast-iron frying pan

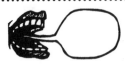

E X P E R T ' S   A D V I C E

Keeping Firewood Dry

Keep your wood dry by spreading a tarp over it at night, or by storing it underneath your picnic table, RV, or car.

directly on the coals. She admitted, however, that she does bring a small backpacker's stove for making coffee in the morning.

Ellen cooks most of their meals in the kitchen of her RV. She has a microwave, a cooktop, and an oven, and she finds it easier and cleaner to cook there. Sometimes they barbecue outside on a propane grill, but never over charcoal or over the fire. Their fire pit is for relaxing conversation.

In between these two extremes, most families cook some foods on a one- or two-burner white gas or propane stove, but almost all want to do some of their cooking on the fire, even if it's only hot dogs on a stick. Michael and Ricki like to find a campsite with a metal barbecue on a post; they cook on charcoal briquettes on the

Building a Fire

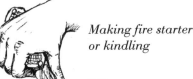

Making fire starter or kindling

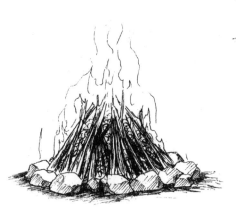

The teepee fire

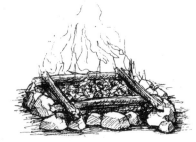

The log house fire

barbecue. Sara's family brings a charcoal hibachi, because, she says, they are "wood-fire challenged."

If you are camping during a very dry season, be sure to check with the local authority on whether there is a burn ban; in that case, campfires will not be allowed and stoves will be required.

Some camping families take pride in the heavy cast-iron pans or the large kettles that have served them well in years of camping. However, these utensils tend to blacken on the outside when exposed to open flames. To keep them cleaner, coat the outside of the pans with soap before using them. The black will wash away

HELPING HANDS

Kitchen Aides

The same kids who might balk at chores in the kitchen at home love to participate in meal preparation outdoors in camp. They will happily wash vegetables or fruit, spread peanut butter or cheese on crackers, or, most fun of all, prepare a meal wrapped in foil.

quickly when you have finished cooking. On the internet, I read of one camper who doesn't wash the outside of his pans until the end of the camping season; he claims that the blacken sides actually absorb heat faster than clean metal.

Bobby and Max, both 12, devoted their entire camping essays to the topic of fire building, with appropriate drawings. Bobby says that starting the fire can be frustrating and difficult. First of all, he advises you to bring a fire starter. Newspaper works well. Max says that if you don't have paper you can shave paper-thin pieces of wood to use as a fire starter, but this is a project for older children. Teach them to put their whole hand on the knife handle, and always cut away from themselves.

Bobby wrote about two shapes of fires, the teepee and the log house. Both start with a wad of crumpled newspaper, but the kindling (thin pieces of wood) laid over the paper will either be in a cone shape or a square shape. If the fire smokes a lot when you light it, Bobby said, it means the wood you brought got wet. If you

Makeshift Grill

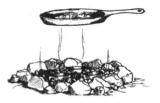

Use two or three tuna cans, with the lids removed from both sides, to hold a big pot in the coals of your fire pit.

camp in a damp area, spread a tarp over your wood pile at night to keep the dew off, or store the wood under your picnic table or car.

As the fire burns, add larger pieces of wood. You can cook over the fire when it burns down to orange or white coals. Max says you should spread the coals so that they are in a waffle shape a couple of inches high so you can put pots or pans on it. Max also suggests getting the flattest stones you can find to use as supports for your pans. Don't use stones from a river, he said, because they might explode from steam built up from the water inside.

My family used the grill, when there was one, but we also carried empty tuna cans, with the lids removed from both sides, to use as emergency pot holders. We stuck the cans in the coals using long-handled tongs, and set the pot on top. For large pans, we used two or three cans.

Keep the fire in the fire pit. Bring a shovel or other tool for managing the fire, and a set of tongs for handling foods in the coals. A spray bottle of water is handy for putting out flames when you don't want them. A bucket of water or sand is useful if the fire gets really out of hand. Warn the kids to stay back from the fire. When you leave the campsite, be sure the fire is totally out and the ashes are cold.

Breakfast

Some families start the day with elaborate preparations of eggs, pancakes, or French toast cooked on a camp stove or campfire, with English muffins or frozen waffles toasted over the fire. Campfire pancakes seem to be a dad specialty in many families. Other families begin the day with oatmeal or other cooked cereals.

Student Isaac, 12, likes Pop Tarts and hot cider or cocoa in the morning when he's too tired to cook.

Three Camp Breakfasts, Easy and Special

1. Pop Tarts and hot cocoa
2. Little boxes of sweetened cereal
3. Individual packets of oatmeal

My friend Vicki, now an adult, remembers eating little boxes of sweetened cereals when she camped as a child, a product she was never permitted at home. Marlene still does the same with her two children, allowing the little boxes only for camping. The Silverman kids ate packets of flavored oatmeal with added raisins, brown sugar, and milk. When they were kids, the milk was powdered; now supermarkets stock Ultra High Temperature (UHT) pasteurized milk, which doesn't need refrigeration until it's opened.

My friend Cathi told me how her Girl Scout troop "scrambles" their breakfast eggs. As the leader, she boils a big pot of water on the fire. The girls each break an egg into a sturdy Ziploc plastic bag and seal it. Actually, Cathi says it's better to break the egg into a small dish and then pour it into the bag—fewer accidents and less mess. With your hands, scrunch the egg around in the sealed

Recipe: Campfire Scrambled Eggs

Crack an egg into a plastic bag and seal it. Use your hands to mush up the egg. Drop the sealed bag into boiling water. Fish it out when it's done. Add condiments of your choice. Eat it from the bag.

baggie until it is the right consistency for scrambling. Drop the bag into the boiling water and leave it until the egg is done.

Cathi sets out omelette-type fixings—chopped vegetables (onions, peppers, tomatoes, mushrooms) and shredded cheese—that she has previously prepared, and the girls add them to their cooked eggs. They eat them straight from the bag. Cathi says it's very important to buy quality baggies that won't rip, and to watch the girls carefully when they drop their eggs into the water and when they fish them out with a tongs or a pierced spoon.

A friend calls this preparation a "Ziploc Omelet." For lunch today, just before I wrote these words, I had a Ziploc omelet. I put chopped green onions, chopped black olives, and chopped mushrooms in a Ziploc bag. Then I broke two eggs into a bowl and poured them into the bag. I sealed it and squished it with my hands to break up the yolk. Then I dropped the bag into a pan of boiling water. The bag wouldn't sink, so I took it out, opened the "zipper" a bit, and pressed most of the air out of the bag. It still wouldn't sink, so I held it under water with a long-handled spoon until the eggs were done. I ate it from the bag. It was delicious.

Lunch

Lunch for many is something that can be carried away from the campsite to the destination for the day. Sandwiches packed in the morning, with everyone gathered around the picnic table making their own, are common. Tuna, peanut butter and jelly, and cheese are favorites. Young Sara, 11, likes turkey and cheddar cheese on a sourdough roll.

Three Easiest Camp Lunches

1. Canned meat spread on Melba toast
2. Meat, cheese, or peanut butter and jelly sandwich
3. Something from a can—chili, macaroni and cheese, or soup

Susan's family eats a big breakfast, so they take snack-type foods for lunch: cheese and crackers, granola bars, nuts, chips, and fresh or dried fruits. My family lunched on Melba toast and canned spreads; we especially liked Underwood brand chicken spread, which my grandson called "devil meat" for the red devil on the label.

Some families who return to their campsite for lunch choose hot dogs or hamburgers. Olivia, 11, says, "It is surprising how different the taste is when it is cooked in the fire rather than in an oven or over a stove." Marlene serves her kids "anything in a can," chili,

Recipe: Pie Iron Sandwich

Take two slices of bread and put something tasty inside, such as peanut butter, cheese, or pie filling. Lightly butter or spray the outside of the sandwich, secure it in the pie iron, and hold it in the fire for two minutes per side, or until the bread is toasted and the filling is heated to your liking.

macaroni and cheese, or soup. Others lunch on instant soup or noodles, reconstituted with hot water.

Christine's mom said that her husband was such a successful fisherman that they always had freshly caught fish for lunch. She enjoys telling the story of how the infant Christine (now grown up) gobbled up fresh trout as fast as they could feed it to her. Stephen, 12, who thinks camping is "one of the funnest things in the world," also eats a lot of fish. He says the fish just "jump on their lines because they like us so much."

The kids who own pie irons—those metal sandwich makers on the end of long sticks—often used them to cook their lunch. You put something that will taste good in a melted form between two slices of bread that has been buttered lightly on the outside. Put the sandwich in the pie iron and hold it in the fire.

Ali, 12, made pizza in hers, by adding sauce, cheese, and "whatever else." Derrick, 11, puts apple pie "stuffing" and cinnamon in his. Peanut butter works, and so does precooked bacon, cheese, and tomato. The kids had different names for the finished

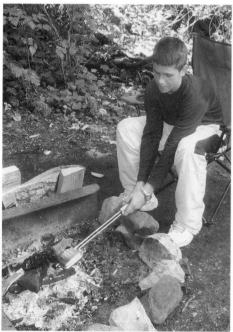

A pie iron is the perfect campfire tool to toast a sandwich.

product: Maddy, 12, called them "roasted star bursts," Mike, 11, called them "dough boys, and their teacher called them "pudgy pies."

The directions that came with my pie iron say that bread should be buttered on the outside, but we found that a spritz of olive oil or non-stick spray worked just fine. The sandwiches toasted quickly—two minutes per side seemed to be sufficient. We especially liked peanut butter with chocolate chips; it was like eating a Reese's cup sandwich.

Dinner

Dinner in camp brings out the most creative cookery. Sarah's family makes shish kebob; they all stand around the table, threading meat and vegetables on long metal skewers before cooking them over the fire. Janelle likes corned beef hash, a recipe she learned

One for Every Day of the Week: Seven Camp Dinners

1. Shish kebob
2. Foil packet stew
3. Grilled steak or chicken
4. Hot dogs
5. Corned beef hash
6. Spaghetti with canned or homemade sauce
7. Canned chili over instant rice

Note that we use the fresh ingredients first, to avoid spoilage, and save pantry supplies for later in the week.

from her father; she brings cooked potatoes from home, shreds them in camp, mixes them with shredded canned corned beef and onion, and cooks them over the fire in a big iron frying pan. The final touch is a fried egg on top.

In her RV kitchen, Ellen re-heats gourmet meals like rotisserie smoked duck or salmon from the deli section of the grocery; she says that trays from Costco just fit in the fridge in her RV. Madelaine's husband grills flank steak or chicken breasts that have been marinating in a plastic bag in the cooler. Henk starts from home with frozen chicken breasts; by the time he is ready to grill them, they are thawed. (Grilling meat seems to be a man's job, even in camp!)

Jeff, 11, and his family often have spaghetti for dinner. After the noodles have cooked in boiling water, he and his brother test them for doneness by throwing cooked noodles at each other; if they are done, he said, "They stick when you throw them at your brother."

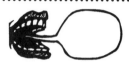

E X P E R T ' S   A D V I C E

The Noodle Test

To test whether their spaghetti noodles are cooked, Jeff and his brother have developed the following method: Throw them at each other. If they are done, "They stick when you throw them at your brother," Jeff said.

Some families bring homemade sauce in their coolers, but many eat their spaghetti with bottled sauce. Sara, 11, said she likes pasta with just cheese, no sauce.

Hot dogs cooked over the fire are probably the simplest supper. Ricki's group brings canned chili and sauerkraut to put on their hot dogs, in addition to mustard and ketchup—chili dogs. Others wrap the cooked hot dog with Bisquik or refrigerated biscuits, and toast them over the fire a second time. But remember, if you cook hot dogs and/or marshmallows, bring sticks or skewers from home. Don't destroy the environment by cutting sticks from growing plants.

Kate's family likes "easy meals," like Lipton's instant rice or noodle combinations that can be cooked in one pan. Diana agrees; she cooks boil-in-the-bag rice and tops it with canned chili. These dishes that use dry ingredients from the pantry are good choices for later in the week; use your fresh ingredients first.

Henk Jr. calls chips and salsa "convenience foods." At my supermarket, looking for convenience foods appropriate for camping, I walked down the aisle marked "Prepared Food" and "Box

Dinners." There, I saw a variety of potential camp dinners based on rice and beans or pasta or potatoes, by Lipton, Rice-a-Roni, Banquet, and Kraft. I also saw turkey, chicken, tuna, and salmon in cans and in foil packages.

Just be sure to read the directions before you buy. Unless you're in an RV, the dinner you choose should be intended for stove-top cooking and not the oven, and it should not require a lot of additional ingredients that you may not have with you. On the other hand, if you select a dinner like pasta with broccoli, you may want to add extra broccoli or chicken to the pan.

Foil Dinners

There is a long list of things you can wrap in foil and roast in the coals. Young Sarah, 9, says her mom bakes potatoes at home in the microwave, and then wraps them in foil and warms them in the fire. You could heat ears of corn the same way. Corn and potatoes are old standbys, but the hands-down favorite dinner of most of the kids I talked to was campfire or foil packet stew. Kids can participate in much of the preparation for this dish—older siblings can cut vegetables, while younger ones can wash them or separate onions into rings.

Recipe: Foil Packet Stew

Lay all your stew ingredients—meat, vegetables, sauce, and/or seasoning—in the middle of a big sheet of heavy-duty aluminum foil. Wrap it securely in a drugstore wrap. Lay it on the coals for 15 minutes, then turn and cook 15 minutes more. Open carefully. Eat it directly from the foil.

Stephanie described for me the way she and her husband and their five kids stand around the picnic table, everyone preparing his or her own dinner. The fun of having this dinner, she said, is the hands-on preparation. The other fun part is opening the package and eating directly out of the foil.

Here's what you do: Start with a big sheet of heavy-duty aluminum foil or doubled regular foil, either way with the shiny side up. Lay a portion of meat (ground beef, ground turkey, sausage, or small chunks of chicken, sausage, or beef) —or, if you're a vegetarian, tofu or vegetables—on the foil. You can pre-mix the ground meat with diced onion if everyone likes onion, but if not, add the onion later. You can also pre-cook and refrigerate the meat at home, so that you're sure it's thoroughly cooked and not raw when the package is opened.

Layer thinly cut vegetables over the meat—carrots, zucchini, onion, garlic, mushrooms, and some kind of starchy vegetable, either white or sweet potatoes or instant rice (don't use regular rice; it won't cook fast enough). Stephanie buys lots of frozen vegetables to add—packages of broccoli, peas, and cauliflower. She said the vegetables are thawed but still cold when they come from the cooler. She also uses frozen pre-cooked potato balls, tater tots, because fresh potatoes take too long to cook. Add a seasoning of your

Foil Packet Cooking

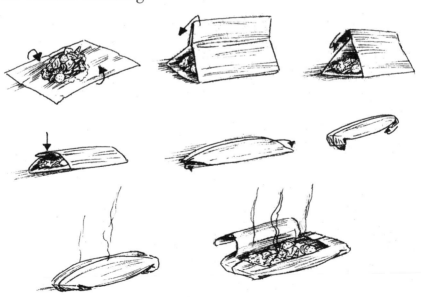

Follow these eight easy steps to make a foil packet.

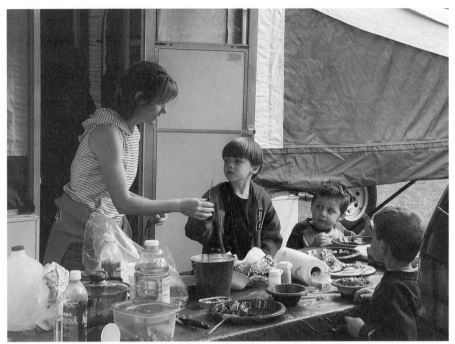

Food is so good in camp, even fussy eaters are satisfied.

choice, like ketchup, mustard, chili sauce, salsa, a little salt or pepper or Worcestershire sauce. Stephanie's family sprinkles one of the dry sauce mixes, taco seasoning or soup mix, over the food; the moisture from the meat and vegetables reconstitutes the sauce.

Wrap the stew packet carefully in a drugstore wrap so it won't leak: Bring the longer edges of the foil together and fold them down several times until you reach the food; then fold the ends over and over until they also reach the food. Some families carry a marking pen so they can initial each packet and identify it after cooking. Others devise a system of creative folding: My packet has two curled corners, his has only one, someone else has turned his corners under or twisted them upwards. But Stephanie says identifying is never a problem in their family because her husband tends the packets in the fire and he always knows which one belongs to whom.

Jack makes a pocket instead of a packet. He lays one sheet of foil over the other, and crimps three sides tightly so he can place the food in the open end. Then he closes the fourth side. I saw a roll of foil pockets in the supermarket in the same section where the other foil rolls were shelved; this new product may or may not be available where you live.

However you prepare it, carefully place each package on the grill or directly on the coals and cook for about 15 minutes. Turn the packets over and cook 15 minutes more. Some children will have difficulty waiting such a long time for their dinner, so their parents bring carrot and celery sticks, tomatoes, cucumbers, and pickles to nosh on while the stews cook.

The foil packets come with warnings. When you settle down to eat, Jessica, 12, says, be careful of the juices that could have developed in the foil, because they are very hot. One of the students told me he got sick from eating a foil-wrapped dinner, so be sure the food is thoroughly cooked. Eleven-year-old Jack's packet once exploded in the fire; maybe he had crimped it too tightly or left it in the fire too long. Fortunately, no one was hurt. Jack's friend tried to grab his packet from the fire and burned his hand, so Jack warns that you always pick it up with something other than your hand.

Other Dinners

When Marlene's family camps, they usually join several other camping families. On one night, they always have a theme dinner, where everyone brings something to share. When it was bouillabaisse night, everyone brought a different kind of seafood to add to the big pot. On pasta night, one person cooked a big pot of noodles, and the rest of the group had a pasta sauce competition. Build-your-own dinners are another popular choice for kids, especially those too young to cut and slice ingredients. Taco salad is fun. A parent browns ground beef on the fire or on one burner of the camp stove and heats canned beans next to them. Each person then layers taco chips, shredded lettuce (washed, dried, and shredded at home, and packed in a sealed plastic bag), grated cheese, chunks of tomatoes, beans, and beef on top. Gourmet cooks can bring sour cream and guacamole in their ice chests. Vegetarians can make the salad without beef.

Kim's family developed a dinner they called "the Mountain." They start with a serving of reconstituted mashed potatoes on each plate and top it with browned ground beef. Then they add chopped vegetables such as onion, mushrooms, tomatoes, or green pepper, and cover the mountain with sauce from a mix—brown or mushroom gravy, cheese, or Stroganoff. Kim likes her mountain all mixed together, but the kids who don't like their foods all mixed up are able to have separate piles of each on their plates.

Michael likes to make stew in a Dutch oven. He combines meat, vegetables, rice (not instant), and a sauce of some kind in the deep pot and sets it on a bed of glowing charcoal briquettes. Then he puts the lid on the Dutch oven, and heaps more burning charcoal on top. A few hours later, he carefully lifts the lid with a special stick that has a hook on the end, so no ashes fall into the stew. Michael says that you can stack Dutch ovens, one on top of the other, with the biggest on the bottom, and cook several courses at the same time.

Dessert

Fresh fruits are a common camping dessert, with watermelon, oranges, berries, and cherries high on the list. Marlene washes the fruit at home before she packs it in the cooler. I find that grapes, washed and pulled from their stems, stay fresh for several days in the cooler in a wide-mouth plastic jar.

Foil packet desserts often follow foil packet dinners. Apple or pear or peach halves sprinkled with brown sugar, nuts, and raisins, are wrapped and cooked on the coals just like the

Ten Favorite Kids' Camp Desserts

1-5. S'mores, OK, but after that, what else?

6. Fresh fruit

7. Banana boats

8. Apples baked in foil

9. Fruit cobbler

10. Hand-cranked ice cream

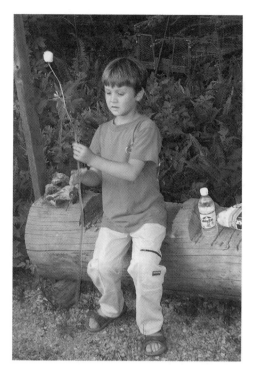

In s'mores, half the goodness is roasting the marshmallow.

stew, except for a much shorter time, only 5 or 10 minutes. On the internet, I read about sugared strawberries baked in foil on the coals; any berries would probably do.

Ava, 11, wrote that her favorite camping food is "jelly dough boys," biscuit mix or refrigerated biscuits wrapped around a stick, toasted in the fire, and filled with jam, jelly "or anything else you can think of!"

Olivia, 11, likes banana boats. She slices the banana the long way, halfway through the center, right through the peel. Then she opens it up and puts inside whatever she chooses. Some things that taste good, she says, are caramel sauce, chocolate sauce, strawberry sauce, nuts of any kind, marshmallows, peanut butter, or any other fruit. Then she closes the banana and wraps it up in foil. She sticks it in the fire for a few minutes until everything melts and it's ready to eat.

Michael and Ricki showed me the brochure that came with their Dutch oven. In it, I read the following recipe for trail cobbler: 2 cups biscuit mix; 2 cups sugar; 2 cups milk or water; 1 cup margarine; 1 large can of fruit. Combine all the ingredients and cook in the Dutch oven about one hour. It makes about eight 1-cup servings. One cup of margarine sounds excessive to me, and, in fact, Ricki told me that they often use less or even none at all. After all, Ricki said, who measures when they're camping?

Ricki makes much simpler fruit cobblers in their Dutch oven. She lines the Dutch oven with aluminum foil to make it easier to clean, and then puts in it one large or two small cans of fruit with their juice. She sprinkles a whole box of white cake mix over the fruit, dots it with margarine and cinnamon, and puts the lid on. She sets the pot on the coals, heaps more coals on the lid, and waits for 45 minutes. This one also serves eight. Peach cobbler is a favorite, but the recipe works with any canned fruit or any kind of cake mix.

In the freeze-dried food section of the outdoor store, campers found fancier desserts, like raspberry crumble or apple brown betty that require just a little cooking. You may also find freeze-dried ice cream. Have you ever left a carton of ice cream in the freezer so long that it began to turn hard and dry? That's the first step to freeze drying it; the final product is sweet and crunchy.

Ali, 12, remembers making homemade ice cream in an old-fashioned wooden ice-cream maker. Everyone had a chance to crank the handle on the bucket and spin the paddles to make the mix solid. The smallest child should have the first turn at the crank, because as the ice cream freezes, the crank becomes harder and harder to turn.

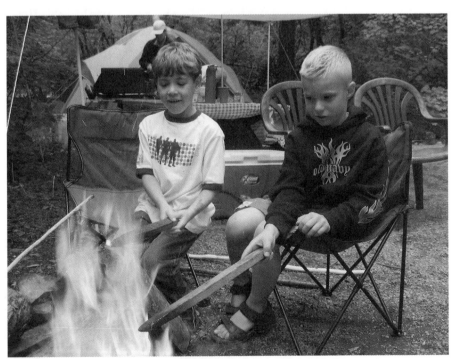

Simple camp pleasures: a comfortable chair, a warm fire, a good friend.

Among the kids I interviewed, the most popular dessert of all has to be s'mores, which Spencer, 11, called "basic American food." Does anyone need instructions for this sandwich of graham crackers, chocolate Hershey bars, and toasted marshmallow? Some kids let their marshmallows catch on fire, to make blackened marshmallows, while others toast them to a golden brown. Randy lays the graham cracker with the chocolate on top of a rock near the fire, so the chocolate begins to melt before the marshmallow hits it. He also suggests substituting a peanut butter cup for the chocolate. When I was a Girl Scout, our leader added a thin slice of apple to our s'mores, to cut the cloying sweetness and make them a little bit more healthy.

When my daughter was a Camp Fire Girl, we learned to make "Angels on Horseback." We cut a loaf of unsliced white bread into chunks 2 inches by 1 inch by 1 inch. We skewered the chunks on our hot dog forks, rolled them first in sweetened condensed milk (not evaporated), and then in shredded coconut. Then we toasted them over the fire. Gooey and sweet, these were delicious.

While the marshmallows or the angels are toasting, many families pop corn over the fire at the same time. The kind that comes wrapped in foil with a wire handle is popular, but Marlene says her family always burns theirs. People in the RVs bring out popcorn that's been microwaved.

Cleaning Up

RV people are lucky. Many have dishwashers. Some tent campers carry two dishpans, one for soapy water and one for rinsing. Others have one basin for all their washing. Either way, they use water heated on the stove or the fire. Campers don't have the luxury of the almost unlimited hot water that they have at home. To keep the dishwater usable, any leftover food on the plates should be thoroughly scraped into the garbage bag and perhaps wiped with a paper towel before they are washed. Sara's family uses paper plates, but they each have their own cup and silverware, which they rinse at the camp water tap.

I was surprised to learn how many people simply carried their dirty dishes to the camp water tap, rinsed them under running water, and called them clean. I think they've been lucky! Dishes should be washed in hot, soapy water and then rinsed in more hot water. Some families put all their washed dishes in a big mesh bag and dip them up and down several times in a deep pot of boiling water. The dirty water should be disposed of properly, either poured out into a designated sink or spilled on bare ground at least 200 feet away from a lake or stream.

Important Cooking Precautions

No one wants to get sick from food, ever, but it's even worse if it happens when you're camping. Make sure your cold foods are kept cold, and that warm or hot foods don't sit around for a long time between warming and eating. Don't prepare foods directly on the surface of the picnic table; use a cutting board and/or disposable cutting sheets. Take the time to boil water to give your dishes and utensils one final rinse. Make sure that your children have clean hands when they handle foods, especially raw meats, and that they wash their hands thoroughly after handling raw meats. Use a hand sanitizer in addition to soap. If you're in a primitive camp, where you're taking water from a lake or stream, it is most important to filter, boil, or treat water for drinking and all cooking and cleaning up afterward. Do not rely on the water supply, even if it may look clear.

What Should We Do for Fun?

I asked every parent I talked to, how do you keep your kids occupied in camp?

Henk Jr. answered immediately, "Oh, that's easy. Just invite another family with kids to go with you." The children enjoy each other's company so much, he said, that they don't need toys, games, or planned activities to keep them happy. The other bonus is for the parents, who gain some adult companionship. Randy agreed.

When there are other children around, he said, there is much less need for toys brought from home. Jeannie had a similar response. She said that often while her husband fished, she walked through the campground looking for kids the same age as Christine, so they could play together.

A Quiet-Time Project

Create a journal together of what you did in camp, written and illustrated by the whole family. Illustrate it with photos or drawings, or capture the whole thing on video.

But while playing with other kids is fun, spending special time with parents, especially for younger children, is also important. Once your camp is set up, or on the second day of your stay, you can begin helping your children create their own fun, using the resources and materials of your campground. Help them learn about and appreciate the outdoors and the natural wonders that brought you to the special place where you are camping.

Seven Different Kinds of Fun in Camp

1. Things to do near water
2. Things to do in the woods
3. Learning about nature
4. Things to do at night
5. Art in camp
6. Games and toys from home
7. Ranger-organized activities

You may even wish to create a family record of your trip, by writing a journal together of what you did. Your younger children who aren't writing yet can dictate what they want you to write for them, and the kids can illustrate the journal by drawing pictures. If you have a camera—film, digital, or video—you can make a photo documentary of your trip. This project could occupy a quiet time after lunch or dinner, or while sitting around the campfire. Bring a notebook, paper, pens, and colored pencils to camp, so you are prepared.

The students who wrote essays about camping for me did a lot of hiking and swimming and building forts and sand castles and rafts and sailboats. In my local library, I found many books with great suggestions for outdoor fun and activities in nature for kids. My favorite was *The Kids Nature Book* by Susan Milord. For convenience, I have grouped the ideas I collected into themes: things to do near water, things to do in the woods, learning about nature, things to do at night, art in camp, games and toys from home, and ranger-organized activities.

Things to Do Near Water

If you are camping near water, use that as your playground. If you are at a beach, children can spend many hours with found objects—collecting shells, stones, bits of glass polished by the sea, seaweed, or driftwood in funny shapes. Filling and emptying a bucket of sand or water is fun. Older children, with their parents' help, can build water courses or sand castles or driftwood forts. It's fun to bury someone in sand, if that person doesn't mind. You can also make a sculpture of a person lying down, and give it eyes and buttons made of shells or stones.

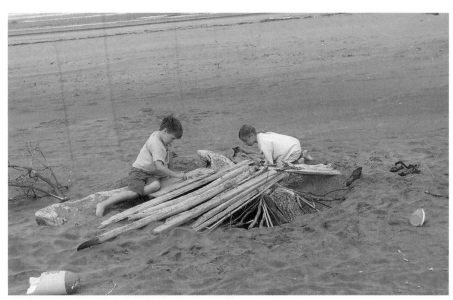

Someone dug a "basement" for this beach house.

If you're camping at an ocean beach, or at a lake big enough to have tides, you can study the high and the low tides. Look for a line along the beach that shows the last highest tide, and examine the debris that the water left behind. If you're at the beach at high tide, mark the highest point with a stick driven into the sand or a line of rocks or shells; return later in the day to see how the tide is ebbing. (You can do a reversal, too. Mark the low tide, and then come back to see how the rising tide has covered your marker.) If your kids are old enough to read a tide table, pick one up before you get to camp and teach your kids how to use it.

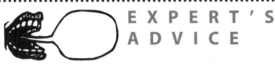

E X P E R T ' S A D V I C E

Fun Near Water

Keep your kids entertained for hours at the beach with these activities:

▶ Collecting shells, stones, beach glass, and driftwood

▶ Filling and emptying buckets of sand or water

▶ Building forts, sand castles, or sculptures

▶ Studying high and low tides

▶ Building sailboats

▶ Creating an underwater viewer

Rocks mixed with water equals fun. I remember camping with my grandchildren near a stream in Mt. Rainier National Park. They filled a small pail with rocks on one side of the stream, crossed the water on a flattened log, and dumped the rocks on the other side of the stream, over and over again.

Years earlier, my kids built sailboats by using a twig "mast" to fasten a leaf to a flat piece of bark. We poked a hole in the bark so the twig would stand up; then we threaded a leaf through the twig to make a "sail." We sailed our boats down little streams or launched them on lakes to see how far they would go.

Sometimes we dropped a stick off the upstream side of a bridge and ran to the other side to see how fast it came through. If someone in your party knows how to skip rocks, that is a challenging skill to pass on to the next generation.

Susan Milord's book included instructions for making an underwater viewer: You need a half-gallon milk carton, clear plastic wrap, and a rubber band or some tape. Cut the top and the bottom off the milk carton. Stretch the plastic wrap over the bottom of the carton, and use the rubber band or the tape to hold it tightly in place. Lower the viewer into the water and put your face in the open end of the carton. The view you get of the lake or stream bottom is the same view you would get through a snorkeler's mask, but you don't get your face wet. If you're not planning to bring cartons of milk or juice to camp, making the viewer could be an at-home project to get the kids excited about going camping.

Things to Do in the Woods

A hike in the woods is a fun activity for kids if it's not too long or boring. I didn't say "not too hard." A hike that involves some kind of challenge, like scrambling up a trail on rocks and roots, or stepping through a patch of mud on planks or rocks, is more entertain-

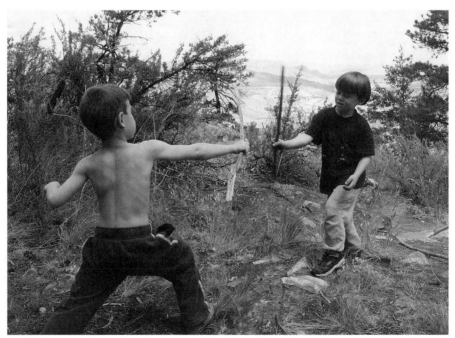

Play in the woods is easy with found "swords" for a duel.

ing than walking on a simple trail. Just walking on a trail can be made to be absorbing, especially for small children, who will find a lot to see on a brief hike. They see flowers and insects and rocks, down at their level, which adults might overlook.

Turning a rock over will reveal all sorts of interesting life. If you are hiking in snake country, choose the rock carefully. Find one in a clear space that is not surrounded by thick greenery. An adult should tap gently around the rock, to be sure that it isn't home to a rattlesnake.

Fun in the Woods

▶ Hiking

▶ Looking under rocks

▶ Looking up into trees

▶ Collecting for a "museum"

▶ Climbing trees

Carry a magnifying glass so you can look at the underside of leaves and ferns, or study the track of ants going to and from their ant hill. Look up in the trees for birds' nests; use binoculars to really see up in the trees. Look at the birds, too. How many different kinds of birds can you see? What colors are they?

Teach your child that flowers and leaves that are attached to a plant should be left alone, but rocks and cones and fallen leaves can be collected. A rock that's turned over should be turned back; the underside is home to many creatures. If a small child has a little bag, he or she can collect all sorts of fascinating things to bring back to your campsite, where they can be laid out in a "museum." At the end of your stay in camp, scatter the collection so the next child who camps in that space can start anew.

Don't expect your child to cover great distances on first hikes. For longer hikes, Randy keeps his 6-year-old daughter going with "power pills," their name for Skittles or M&Ms. Small candies and raisins make good incentives for young hikers. To avoid choking accidents, come to a complete stop for these treats, and be sure they have been swallowed before you move on.

Hiking isn't the only thing to do in the woods. Two Sarahs I know love climbing trees. When I met Isbela and Oscar at a US Forest Service camp, they were up in a big tree near their campsite.

Learning About Nature

The beach, the woods, a big grassy area—any of these places is a laboratory for learning about nature, except that your children will think they are playing.

Get up early, or stay up late, to watch the sun rise and set, and the moon do the same. Have the children follow the track of the sun across the sky, over the course of a day. They can note where it rises and where it sets, where it is at breakfast and where it is at lunch. The shadows at your campsite will change; the kids can mark the end of the shadows at different times of day. Then you can talk to them about whether the sun and moon are really moving, or whether from our observation point on earth we just think they move.

Six Ways to Study Nature's Mysteries

1. Observe the sun and the moon

2. Study the clouds

3. Use the sun to heat water

4. Condense salt from salt water

5. Make a bird nest

6. Look at bugs

Find an open space where your whole family can lie down and look at the clouds. Encourage everyone to find shapes in the clouds. Parents should prepare ahead of time, so you can recognize the different cloud formations, and explain to your children the difference between a cirrus and a cumulous cloud.

Use the sun to heat water. This is a great experiment for kids. Have them put some water in a clear plastic baggie or in an open white container, and put the same amount of water in a black container. If you don't have a black container, wrap a black garbage bag around your water container. Leave the containers out in the sun together, and after a few hours, check to see which one holds

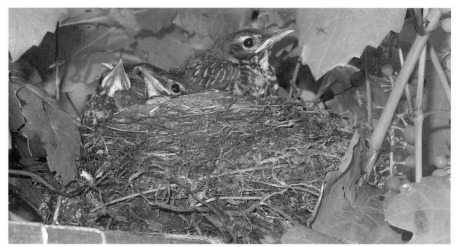

If you see a bird nest, have your kids look at it—but not touch it—and then try to build their own.

hotter water. Don't tell the kids which container will hold hotter water; let them find out for themselves.

If you're camping near salt water, your kids can condense salt from the sea. If they have a few days, have them fill a container with salt water and let it sit in the sun; if you have only a short stay, have them evaporate the water by carefully placing it in your campfire. Let everyone taste the salt water before and after, and then talk to your kids about the way people all over the world create their own salt by removing it from the sea.

Another idea from Susan Milord: Have your children build a bird nest, just the way a bird would do it. If you find a bird nest, you can all study it carefully. If not, remind the kids that birds don't pick living plants, so have them collect fallen plant materials such as twigs, grass, and leaves, and have them use mud to put a nest together. Then have them find some pretty egg-shaped rocks to go in the nest.

Look at bugs. Help the kids capture a few in a jar with holes punched in the lid so the creature can breathe, and study it. What can they see? Note the colors, the legs, whether it has wings, eyes, antennae. Try to identify what they have found. The visitors centers at some large parks have information about the wildlife in the park, including the bugs. If there's a ranger, sometimes he or she will know what kind of bugs you have found. Maybe the children would like to keep a record of the bugs they find, either by writing in a journal or by drawing a picture or taking its picture. In any case, when they have finished looking at the bug and before it perishes, return it to the area where they found it. Teach your children that they can observe the natural world without being destructive.

Things to Do at Night

In the lights of the city, the moon and especially the stars are lost to view. In a campground, far away from city lights, the number of stars is amazing. If your children can stay awake that late, just gazing at the stars and the moon is fantastic. Younger children can share your amazement at the myriad numbers of stars in the sky. Older children can begin to recognize some of the constellations. You can talk to them about the phases of the moon, whether it is waxing or waning. If there happens to be a meteor shower during the nights you are camping, you can all find an area with a clear view of the sky, lie on your backs, and count the "shooting stars."

Four Things to Look for at Night

1. The moon
2. The stars
3. Meteors
4. Night-flying bugs

How, you may be asking, does she expect me to know what the moon is doing or when to look for meteors? I'll tell you. One of my favorite websites is www.stardate.org, which is administered by the University of Texas McDonald Observatory. It tells you exactly what is happening in the sky every night for the month; you can also look at the sky of other months. You and your children can visit the site before you leave home, so you'll know what to look for when you're camping. You can look up the months when your children were born and show them the sky at that time. They can learn a lot about space and astronomy at that site, and so can you.

The McDonald Observatory also does a brief presentation called StarDate on National Public Radio; consult your local station for times.

But don't spend all your time looking at the stars. There are other things to do at night. Have the children look for night creatures. You may not see any animals; they're pretty shy. But moths may be attracted to your bright lantern, and you can talk to the kids about the difference between moths and butterflies. (Look at the way moths hold their wings when they land; the next day, look at a butterfly at rest. There's a difference. Moths spread their wings out flat when they rest, while butterflies hold them up vertically.) If you're lucky enough to be camping in a place that has fireflies, let the kids capture one very gently in a jar just to look at it; then let it go.

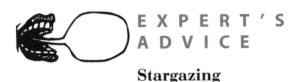

E X P E R T ' S   A D V I C E

Stargazing

Visit www.stardate.org to learn about the night sky.

Here's one more scientific experiment to do in the dark. When you pack your camp snacks, toss in a package of wintergreen mints or LifeSavers. Then when it's dark at your campsite, douse all the lights so that it's really dark, put a mint between your teeth and chomp down on it. There will be a blue flash. Perhaps you should have mirrors handy, so everyone can see his or her own flash. This may not work with other kinds of mint, so be certain to bring wintergreen.

Art in Camp

In a quieter moment, children can use the items they have collected to create art objects in camp. Someone needs to prepare for these projects before you leave home. The children can help plan and pack the art materials, so they can look forward to doing the projects in camp, or you can surprise them with the activity in camp. Bring out the glue, construction paper, string, paints, and other materials and let nature inspire your creativity!

Raina's daughters make collages of neat things they find—twigs, small cones, fallen leaves, ferns, rocks, sand, and beach glass. Your kids can do that, or they can make a wind chime from shells, beach glass, and driftwood. Use glue and bits of string from home, but if the kids have found string on the beach, they might prefer to use that. Bring little cardboard boxes like jewelry or pill boxes that they can cover with glued-on shells or stones. Have them make picture frames by gluing flat pieces of driftwood into a rough rectangle, and then gluing the shells and stones to that. Later they can put their own pictures in the frames.

C H E C K L I S T

Art Materials to Bring from Home

▶ Glue

▶ Construction paper

▶ String

▶ Paint (watercolors and poster paint)

▶ Paint brushes

▶ A roller

▶ Colored pencils

▶ Cotton balls

▶ Plain white paper

With a stack of paper, a roller, and a jar of poster paint, the kids can make block prints of some of these found objects. Dip the roller in the paint, run it over the object, and then press the object down on a piece of paper. Older kids can also make prints using half of a potato, with a design carved into it, under adult supervision. Dip the potato in paint and then press it onto paper. Younger kids can make prints using an apple cut in half across the middle (a task for the adult in the group), so that the star pattern shows.

Kids can use the glue you brought (maybe you should bring more than one bottle!) to make a sand picture. If the kids are quite young, you should draw a shape, like an animal or a flower, on a piece of construction paper. Older children can draw their own outlines. Spread glue over the shape. Sprinkle sand over the glue. If you're camping near a beach that has sand in more than one color, the kids can make very interesting pictures. Or you can collect the sand from different beaches and make the sand pictures when they have more than one color to work with.

If you and the children have been looking at clouds, they may want to make cloud pictures. Use cotton balls glued onto sky blue construction paper. If you're been seeing cirrus clouds, pull the cotton balls into sheer wisps and glue them down. For cumulous clouds, glue the puffy balls one on top of the other. Or have the kids create a night sky with dark blue paper and little dots of paint for stars. What kind of moon did they see? They can paint it.

If your children enjoy drawing and painting, have them paint pictures of what they have seen at camp or on their hikes. You can bring paint from home, but it's fun to make your own too. Paint consists of color and a binder, to hold the color together. Tell your children that famous old painters used egg yolks as their binder; it's called egg tempera. There are lots of other liquids that can be binders that they will have in camp—glue, oil, and even water.

The fun part is finding the colors in nature. Have the children look around for material that could be ground up for color. Is there charcoal in the fire pit? Is there ash? After carefully checking that the charcoal and the ash are cold, you can use them to

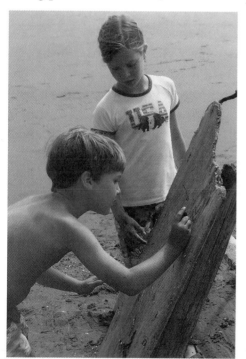

At the beach, your kids may discover their inner van Gogh.

make black and gray. Is the soil at your campsite red or brown? Is there clay nearby? Are there colored rocks? With a big rock or a hammer, help the kids break up the colors that they find and mix them with a binder. Then have them use the paint to create a picture. This is a good time to talk to your children about the cave paintings and pictographs that ancient people left. If there are pictographs near your camp, you may want to visit them first, before you create your own art.

If making paint was fun, try making paint brushes. Use found materials—a leaf, a twig, a piece of seaweed—to create your pictures. If your kids didn't like making paint and brushes, maybe they're

HELPING HANDS

Planning Activities

Encourage the children to decide which activities they would like to do in camp, and let them select and assemble the toys they want to take.

like Raina's daughters, who prefer water colors with fine brushes for painting rocks.

My daughter-in-law Judith suggested that children can make a leaf book in camp. There are a number of ways to use art to transfer the leaf shape to a page. One way is to make a leaf print: Roll poster paint across the underside of the leaf where the veins and stem will show, turn it over, and press it down hard on a piece of paper. Another way is to make a leaf rubbing: Lay the paper over the leaf with the underside up, and rub a crayon or a colored pencil gently back and forth until the leaf shows up. (For rubbings, construction paper may be too thick; if you plan to do rubbings, bring lighter weight paper. Judith suggests buying the cheapest plain paper you can find.)

A third method, and possibly the easiest, is to use the leaf as a stencil: Just lay the leaf on the page, paint around all the edges, and then very carefully lift the leaf so that its shape remains on the paper. Judith suggests that the kids should label each page with the date and the name of the tree from which the leaf came. That's assuming that parents will know the name, or else be able to find it, and that's another project. (If there are rangers in the camp where you're staying, they should be able to help identify the trees.)

Games and Toys from Home

Although some parents rely entirely on found amusements, many bring some toys or games from home. Favorite trucks and cars, for hauling and dumping sand and rocks, are big with small children. Bicycles, scooters, skateboards, roller skates, and tricycles all show up in camps. While most drivers are conscientiously slow driving through the campground, children need to be made aware of traffic on the roads. Parents may want to stay next to small children on tricycles.

Some families recommend a Whiffle ball and bat, a badminton set, or Frisbees. Buckets and shovels are almost necessities at a beach, but if you forget them, use a cup and a spoon. A kite is great at the beach but won't be much fun in a forest camp. If there is a lake near your campground, bring inner tubes or an inflatable boat; if you bring a boat, also bring life jackets. If there is a big lawn, bring a croquet set. If there are tennis courts, bring rackets.

• •

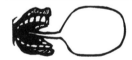

E X P E R T ' S   A D V I C E

Safe Play

Don't forget safety and accessories when packing games and toys. If you bring an inflatable boat or inner tubes for floating, also bring life jackets.

• •

Much depends on the park where you're camping; you are more likely to find tennis courts and lawns in a private park such as a KOA campground, than in a Forest Service camp.

Bring some supplies for quiet times, too: books, art supplies, a tape or CD player with favorite tunes, a portable radio. Lots of people bring cards, and the RV campers also bring board games that the whole family can play. Sandra remembers playing cards by flashlight in her family's tent. Alaina and her kids, Isabela and

Oscar, play tic-tac-toe and checkers with candy; any time a player jumps a man, he gets to eat him.

A camera is also fun for kids. If you have a digital camera, you can delete the pictures of sky or feet that your children take, and print one or two of their better camp pictures. Children can frame their pictures in the picture frames they made from their found materials. If the kids aren't fast enough to capture a bird or an animal with the camera, they can draw a picture of the creature with simple colored pencils or felt-tip pens and plain paper. Wendy says that colored pencils are better than crayons, because crayons may melt in hot weather.

Although Ellen says her kids take "everything they own" in their RV, too many toys can become a nuisance. RVs with more storage area have the advantage over tents with limited space. Bridgit's RV has a "basement," a storage area under the coach. She packs toys in plastic storage tubs and rotates them every few days, so the coach interior doesn't fill with clutter. A tent will fill with toys even more quickly. Nevertheless, if a child is really attached to certain toys, and especially if she is a somewhat reluctant camper, it's a wise idea to find room in the tent for her Barbies.

You may be thinking that all these activities represent a lot of work for parents, and they would if you did everything for every trip and did all the selecting and packing yourself. But this is a good area for input from the kids. Let them have a voice in what they would like to take camping, and what they would like to do in camp. Especially after the first time, they may have definite ideas on how to spend their time. Do give them some guidance; Wendy says that toys taken on trips should be big, solid toys; leave the Lego at home.

Ranger-Organized Activities

Not all the activities in camp need to be parent-directed. Most larger campgrounds, especially at state and national parks, will have rangers who may lead guided walks during the day and give talks in the evening. Though they are sometimes called "campfire talks," there is usually not a campfire, but an informative and often funny conversation between rangers and visitors. If there is a visitors center, there may be lectures and presentations there.

I've saved the best for last. A ranger at Haleakala National Park in Hawaii told me about the Official Junior Park Ranger program of the National Park Service, and he gave me the activity booklet for that park. The next day, at Hawaii Volcanoes National Park, I picked up a different booklet. When I got home, I made a few phone calls and surfed the internet, and I learned that some state parks also have a Junior Ranger Program. Before I stopped search-

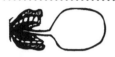

E X P E R T ' S   A D V I C E
Junior Rangers

Check with the ranger at your state or national park campground for the Junior Ranger Activity Book. You can also look on the internet and order activity books in advance. Your child can become an Official Junior Ranger by taking part in age-appropriate activities in the park.

ing, I found the program in Washington, Oregon, California, Colorado, and Wisconsin. I now own a neat stack of activity books for kids. Even the Washington State Ferries has an activity book.

Each park that participates in this program has a booklet of its own listing age-appropriate activities for kids in that park. The activities help children learn more about the natural world of the park and also about proper park behavior, like staying on trails and not disturbing wildlife. Booklets vary, because each park's staff prepares the booklet for that facility. Sometimes the booklet is free, and in other parks there is a small fee. When a child has completed the prescribed number of activities, he or she can report to a ranger at park headquarters to take the Junior Ranger Pledge and receive a Junior Ranger badge and certificate.

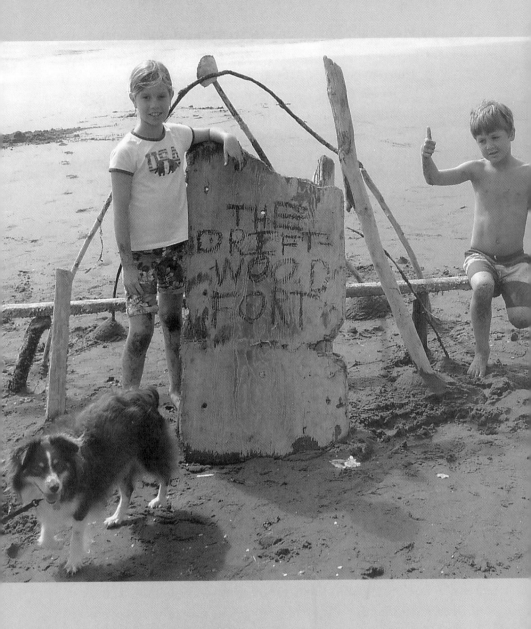

Staying Safe, Sound, and Happy

▶ What Contingency Plans Should We Make?

▶ How Do We Stay Safe on the Road?

▶ What Are the Dangers in Camp?

▶ What Basic First Aid Do We Need to Know?

▶ What if Someone is Lost?

It would be wonderful if all camping experiences were happy days spent eating great meals outdoors, exploring, learning to love the outdoors, and carrying out fun projects with the whole family working together. Unfortunately, it doesn't always happen that way. Some of the people I talked to told me of experiences that were less than happy. Sometimes things go wrong, and the most grown-up people in the family have to guide the rest of the group through the situation.

What Contingency Plans Should We Make?

When my children were young, our catchphrase for camping was, "Be flexible." If the toast fell on the ground, butter side down, we said, "Be flexible," brushed it off, and ate it. If it rained the weekend we planned to camp, we said, "Be flexible," and drove to the dry side of the mountains. Campers in western Washington state do that all the time; we know that when it's raining on our side of the Cascade Range, it will probably be dry on the eastern side. In the back of our minds, we always have a plan B, a contingency, in case the trip we have planned doesn't work out the way we want it to.

Contingency planning is another opportunity for imaginary camping. Not to be morbid, but think about some of the things that might go wrong on your trip, and in your imagination walk through the steps you would take in that situation. Besides bad weather, you might think of not getting into the park of your choice, forgetting some important supplies, someone getting sick, or an automobile breakdown.

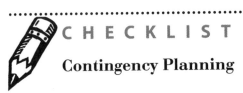

CHECKLIST
Contingency Planning

Things you should know about the area you're visiting:

▶ What are the local tourist sights?

▶ Where is the nearest grocery store?

▶ Where is the nearest gas station?

▶ Where is the nearest hospital?

A contingency plan might begin with some research on where you are going. Find out what the tourist sights are, in case the camping isn't working. Is this area historically significant? Are there sites to visit? Is there some natural wonder nearby, like a cave, that you can visit even when it's raining?

You should also make note of the nearest grocery store, gas station, and hospital. If you are renting an RV, be sure you know what to do in event of a mechanical problem.

Contingency planning or being flexible often involve thinking about weather. A rainy day in a weeklong campout could be a reason for packing up and going home, but if they're prepared for the possibility of bad weather, many campers stick it out, waiting for better days. Campers in RVs have the advantage once again: They read, play games, listen to music, raid the refrigerator. If the park has a visitors center, a rainy day is a good time to make an in-depth visit. A walk in the rain, bundled into good rain gear, followed by a return to hot chocolate in the cozy RV can be a pleasant camping memory. Tent campers can do almost all those things. Preparing meals under a dining fly will be a greater challenge, but as long as the family has proper clothing and a tent that doesn't leak, a rainy day in camp can be a challenge and not a disaster.

Six Things to Do on a Rainy Day

1. Read
2. Play games
3. Listen to music
4. Snack
5. Walk in the rain
6. Go into the nearest town

If spending a day rained in at your campsite seems just too gloomy to endure, you can always visit the nearest town. Many campgrounds are located close to small towns that may have all sorts of attractions. Look for local museums or interesting shops selling the local artifacts. If all else fails, you can go to the movies.

Campers who go out without reservations also have to be flexible and have a contingency plan. When some parties were too late to find a spot at Jesse M. Honeyman State Park in Oregon, the gatekeepers sent them down the road to a county park. That alternate park wasn't right on the sand dunes, but the campers there were flexible enough to drive to the state park every day and take advantage of the facilities as day users.

When we met Eliot, 8, and his grandfather at a campground near Seattle, they asked us about the nearest town where they could go grocery shopping. They had left one bag of supplies behind. Driving into town to shop also is being flexible.

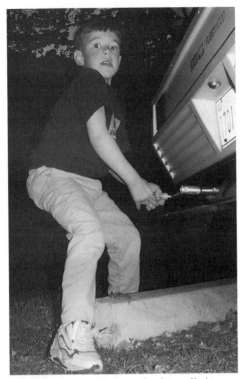

Some kids must be watched at all times.

If someone in the family gets sick, you have a hard decision to make. When my husband's back went out on a weekend backpack, the children and I left him lying on his air mattress while we hiked to a higher lake for the day. The next day, we parceled out most of the gear in his pack into other packs, and he was able to walk out. However, most sick people feel more comfortable in familiar surroundings. A sick child could be a reason for cutting short a trip; a really sick or injured child could be a reason for stopping at the nearest emergency room.

Bryn, 11, learned about emergencies and to "always have one eye on my little sister" after a game of follow the leader. In a class essay assignment, Bryn wrote, "I scurried across a log above a small creek, and my sister followed me. When I jumped off the log, I made sure to jump over the sharp limb that was sticking out at the side. I thought that I had better tell my sister, because I did not want her to miss it and hurt herself... I turned around, but I was too late." The whole family left camp and rushed off to the nearest emergency room, two hours away, where doctors removed wood splinters and stitched up her sister's leg. After an overnight at a hotel, they returned to their campsite the next day, packed up, stopped at the hospital once again so doctors could check the wound, and went "back to our normal life," Bryn wrote.

Finally, you should always let someone at home know that you are going away. This can be a family member or a neighbor. Tell them where you are going and what alternative plans you have made in case your original plans don't work out. Tell them when you will return, too, so that they can call out the searchers if you have a mishap and can't get home. And be sure to call them when you do get home.

If you're going to be away for many days, arrange to have someone take in your mail and newspapers, so your home doesn't present an unoccupied look to potential thieves. If you have plants that need tending, arrange to have someone do that, too. In fact, it's a wise idea to have someone check your vacant house periodically to make sure nothing has happened there, like the flood from the leaking water heater that greeted two of my friends when they came home from their vacation.

Sometimes being flexible means preparing alternate plans, and at other times it means having flexible attitude. Cindy told me that a group of friends, including 5-year-old Michael and 4-year-old Justin, were at the headwaters of the Mississippi River, a creek so narrow that they could wade across. Of course, the little boys did just that. When they came out of the water, Michael discovered that he had a leech clinging to his leg. Nobody gasped or screamed, but the two mothers, in Cindy's words, "tried to keep a straight face," and commented that this was a very interesting creature. Michael was thrilled. He jumped around saying, "I'm Leech Man, I'm Leech Man, look at me!" Justin was upset because when the adults examined him closely he didn't have any leeches, but they did find some mosquito bites, so they dubbed him "Mosquito Man" and that seemed to satisfy him.

Cindy didn't tell me whether she was horrified when she saw the leech on her son. I know I would be, but by maintaining their straight faces and not panicking, the adults showed the children how to react. It should go without saying that children will look to their parents for cues on how to act when they are in a strange situation.

How Do We Stay Safe on the Road?

Comfort and fun are important considerations when you're making vacation plans, but there's an even more important and often neglected concern—safety. Accidents happen, but with a little forethought, they can be avoided. If they do occur, you can be prepared to deal with them.

The most dangerous part of your camping trip is the drive to the campsite. Most states have very specific rules about how and where children may ride in a vehicle. Roger Arnell of RV Gold in Oregon told me that he reviews his insurance company's rules on safety with everyone who rents one of his motorhomes. In addition, every state has its own laws about child-safety restraints.

Safety in the Car

In Washington state, where I live, the law is very clear. Babies must be buckled into rear-facing infant seats for as long as they can possibly fit into them. All other children under age 16 must be seated with

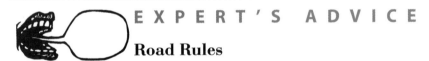

E X P E R T ' S   A D V I C E

Road Rules

Most states have very specific rules about how and where children may ride in a vehicle. Before you leave home, learn the rules for your state and the states where you'll be traveling. If you're traveling in an RV, find out if there are specific regulations for safe travel in a motorhome for your state and the states you will be visiting. Contact the state highway patrol or the governor's office in each state for information.

Kristen Thorstenson of the Washington State Safety Restraint Coalition recommends the five-step test for adjusting a child in a seat belt:

1. The child's bottom must be up against the back of the seat.

2. His or her knees must be able to bend at the edge of the seat.

3. The lap belt must be on the lap, not the tummy.

4. The shoulder belt must be across the chest and shoulder.

5. The child needs to stay that way for the whole trip.

restraints in forward-facing seats. Children under 6 or under 60 pounds must use a car seat. Any other children must be seated either in a booster seat properly attached by lap and shoulder harnesses to a forward-facing seat or else in a properly fastened and adjusted seat belt. Although the rear seat of the family car is much safer, children may be seated in the front seat if there is no other place for the child; however, the front seat is deadly for a child in a crash if there is an air bag.

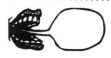

E X P E R T ' S   A D V I C E

Ample Amps?

Take an inventory of the amps of each of the electrical appliances in your RV. This will help you monitor your usage and prevent loss of power.

Nobody sets out on a vacation planning to have a collision, but even a sudden stop can send every loose object in a vehicle crashing forward. Kristen Thorstenson of the Washington State Safety Restraint Coalition warned that unbelted passengers in a sudden stop are "like tennis shoes in a dryer." You want your children to be as safe as you can possibly make them.

Safety in an RV

A lap belt in a forward-facing dinette bench in an RV would *not* meet the law for a child under 6 in Washington. It would meet the letter of the law for a child over 6, but a sudden stop could send that child crashing into the dinette table. The image of a child sitting at a table with a coloring book as the family rolls along is tempting, but for safety's sake the table should be folded down and out of the way. The belts on side-facing couches or rear-facing seats in an RV would not be acceptable for holding car seats or older children in Washington.

Some motorhomes have a second set of swivel chairs behind the driver and copilot. These would be safe for children if they can be locked into a forward-facing position, and if they had shoulder and

CHECKLIST

Before You Drive Off in Your RV

▸ Clear the interior—put everything away.

▸ Turn off propane system.

▸ Check the exterior—door step, bicycles, awning, jacks.

lap belts to hold the car seat in place. Older children and adults in the cabin of the RV could also be belted into forward-facing locked swivel chairs, or in any other forward-facing seats.

Safety in a trailer isn't an issue. No one, adult or child, should be riding in the trailer when it's on the highway. In Washington, an adult over age 16 can ride in a camper truck if all the seats in the front are filled, but children are not allowed to ride in the back of the camper.

In addition to the concerns expressed above, there are other safety considerations for RVs. Certainly a nuisance, if not an immediate safety issue, is a blown electrical circuit breaker. In a flyer from KOA, I read how surprisingly fast the amps can add up to cause your breaker or the RV park's breaker to trip. If your RV has a 30- or 50-amp system, and you start the day by turning on a microwave oven (12.8 amps), an electric coffee maker (9 amps), and a toaster (10 amps), while the refrigerator (5.7 amps) is running, then if someone takes a hot shower (12.5 amps) or turns on the heater (10 amps) or the air conditioner (15 to 17 amps), look out! The flyer suggests that an inventory of the amps of each of your electrical appliances can help you monitor your usage and prevent loss of power.

Another source of anxiety for RVers, just as it can be for all campers, is packing up and getting all the gear in proper order every time you leave camp. The checklist above is a compilation of several lists to use before you depart.

First of all, clear the interior. All counters should be bare, the interior cabinet doors should be closed, and the contents of cupboards and the refrigerator should be secured. That means the soap dish in the bathroom should be put away and every container

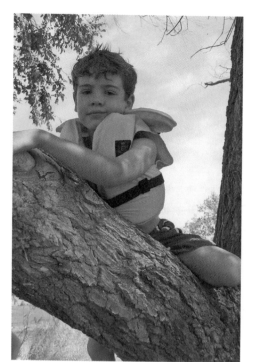

Wearing a life vest is a good safety measure, but it won't save a child stranded in a tree.

in the kitchen and bath should have a tight-fitting lid and be stowed in a cupboard. Objects on upper bunks and couches that might fly off in a sudden stop should be stored. The bathroom door and all other doors should be fastened, either in open or closed position.

The propane system should be turned off. If your RV doesn't have an electrical option for the refrigerator, you need to buy ice to keep the contents cold while you're underway. If you stop for lunch along the road, don't stand in front of the open door while you decide what you want from the refrigerator. Plan ahead and open and close the door quickly.

Check the exterior of your RV before you leave camp. The door step should be up and all the outside compartments closed and locked. Bicycles and other attachments should be securely locked in their racks. The fold-out awning should be rolled up and secure. Leveling jacks should be out of the way. Make sure that your vehicle is properly balanced according to the manufacturer's instructions for on-the-road stability.

If you must back out of the parking area, assign someone to stand behind and watch out for obstacles. That person should watch the top and the sides as well as the back of the vehicle. Trees or low branches could damage the RV.

All mirrors should be adjusted for the driver. The emergency brake should be off, and all occupants should be wearing proper restraints.

What Are the Dangers in Camp?

Children need to be watched carefully in camp, especially around fire, at the beach, and around wild animals, but perhaps the most common potential source of danger is weather.

Weather-Related Problems

Jane and Bill were experienced car campers when they decided to take their three children, ages 5, 7, and 10, to the next level—backpacking. They thought they were planning prudently; they picked a weekend when the weather forecasters promised fair and warm weather, and they replaced their old tent with a new one. The desti-

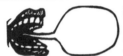

E X P E R T ' S   A D V I C E

Preparing for a Storm

Never rely on a weather prediction. Be prepared for foul weather no matter what the forecasters have said. When you're at camp, even if the evening is calm, ready your campsite for a storm, just in case. Check the stakes and the guy lines of your tent. Dry foods should be in the car or in waterproof containers. Make sure that anything that might blow away is firmly fastened down or stored in the car. Look at the things you've left out and ask yourself, will it survive a heavy onslaught of wind and rain?

nation they chose was only 5 or 7 miles from the trailhead—it was some time ago, and they don't remember that detail, but they remember the rest of their adventure clearly.

After a long day hiking in, they set up camp and prepared to enjoy the weekend. But the weather forecasters were wrong. During the night, it began to rain, and their new tent leaked. They had brought no rain gear or warm clothes because the predictions had been so positive. There was nothing to do but hike out, so at daybreak they started, slogging through the rain that continued all the way. They wrapped themselves in every piece of clothing that they had with them; one of the kids wore underpants on his head in lieu of a hat. Bill carried the youngest most of the way. Jane was convinced that they were not going to make it out. When she saw their car, she burst into tears. Later, she cut the tent up and made it into drawstring bags.

When I asked Bill what he had learned from this experience, he said, "Never trust a weather forecast." He might also have added, check all new equipment before you use it to be sure it works the way it's supposed to.

Derrick, 11, wrote a story about a huge storm that attacked his family's trailer. In the middle of the night, he said, the wind was howling and blowing so hard that the trailer was shaking. Their awning was down, and the wind got under it and ripped it over the top of the trailer. It felt as if they were in a tornado. The next day, another camper told them that his awning had been down also. This man went outside to try to roll the awning up so it wouldn't rip off, and the wind actually lifted him up in the air.

When I talked to Clark Carr of Island RV in Hawaii, he told me that he instructed his rental customers not ever to unroll the awning because, in his experience, the awnings were too easily damaged. Instead, Clark sends them off with a big beach umbrella.

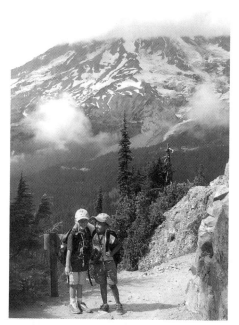

Clouds can roll in quickly in the mountains.

Certainly, one might surmise that it's a wise idea to roll the awning up at night.

Katy, 11, described "the wettest camping trip" she had ever been on. The rain began on the second day, while they were hiking, and they had to put on "ugly plastic ponchos." At lunch time they set up a tarp and huddled together to eat the foods they had packed. Back at their campsite, they dressed in dry clothes, putting on as many layers as they could. They put the tarp up again, but it was "barely big enough for us to sit under in our big, comfy camping chairs." Her father tried to light a fire with wet wood, and then poured stove fuel on the fire, saying to his daughters, "Never do this, girls." The huge flames that shot up lasted only a short time; luckily, no one was burned. The next day, they left for home, a day early. Katy's conclusion: "Now we know to always bring plenty of tarps when we go camping." She might have added, "Never throw stove fuel on a fire."

Accidents in Camp

The conventional definition of an accident may be something "happening by chance," but many mishaps are not accidents at all. It is not an accident, for instance, when someone's behavior is rash and risky. That "accident" is a consequence of unwise behavior. Therefore, the best way to avoid accidents is by practicing safe behavior in camp.

Danger with Fire

The kids in the classes that I talked to told some horrific tales about injuries and near-injuries around fires. You already know, from the cooking section, that foil packages of stew should be lifted out of the fire by some kind of tool and opened carefully to avoid burning steam. You know that a foil packet left in the fire too long could explode, and that flat stones from a river or a stream, placed in the fire to hold a pot or a pan, might explode from steam generated by water trapped inside.

There were other explosion stories. One student told about an exploding TV dinner heated in the fire. Nicole, 12, described how she and her friend were experimenting with methods for cooking clams by placing them on the coals. They left one in the fire too long. "When the clam went KABOOM!!!" she wrote, "some of the little bits of shell and clam gut spattered us." Luckily, no one was hurt.

Bryce, 11, told of a can of FLAMMABLE (his capitals) bug spray left near wood arranged in the fire pit. Not knowing that the bug spray had leaked into the wood, they applied a match, and, Bryce wrote, "BAM! Fire shot out of the wood." Bryce believes that the bug spray itself was flammable, but no aerosol can should be left near the fire.

Some kids were burned by grabbing hold of charred objects that had not cooled off. Carolina, 11, described how she burned her hand grabbing a log to move it when she was "too young to know

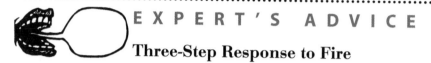

E X P E R T ' S   A D V I C E

Three-Step Response to Fire

If someone's hair or clothing should catch fire, remember to stop, drop, and roll!

how long logs would stay hot." Blackened marshmallows for s'mores can be too hot to handle. Cooked hot dogs should be removed from their sticks very carefully.

The worst imaginable accident around fire would be to have someone's long hair or clothing catch fire. Though none of the people I interviewed knew of such a terrible calamity, I found warning on the web of what to do in such a situation. Teach your children the old slogan, "Stop! Drop! Roll!" The worst action a person could do would be to run. Get the person in flames down on the ground, roll him in bare dirt, and smother the flames with a jacket or a blanket.

A recent article in the *Seattle Times* suggested that we should "extinguish the urge to build a campfire." The author, Terry Wood, an editor at REI, noted the large number of forest fires caused by "escaped campfires," and went on to say that a campfire is not really essential to a legitimate camping experience. Cooking on a stove is cleaner, faster, and safer. If a campfire seems desirable for social reasons, for sitting around of an evening roasting a few marshmallows, it should be a small fire and it should comply with local regulations.

Dangers at the Beach

Jumping around on the dry logs washed up by the highest tides is one of the most fun things to do at the beach. Wading into the cold ocean is a close second. Kelly, 11, was wading when she felt a sharp pain and found a big gash on her foot; her friend said a crab had pinched her, but more likely she had stepped on a piece of broken glass. Unfortunately, broken glass can be found in any lake or stream; too often, we find it when someone steps on it. That's not to say your children shouldn't wade, but an old pair of tennis shoes or a pair of saltwater sandals would be safer than bare feet.

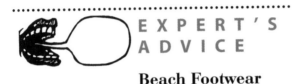

E X P E R T ' S A D V I C E

Beach Footwear

Bring a pair of old tennis shoes or sandals for wading in the ocean or any lake or stream.

One of the most frightening camping experiences of my life occurred at the beach. My husband had put our two young children, 3 and 5 at the time, up on a solitary log that had washed up on the shore, so the incoming waves would not get them wet. A bigger wave came in, rolled the log, and the children fell off. If the log had rolled over them, they would have been pinned in the incoming tide, but it rolled the other way. We grabbed the kids and ran up the beach. Those children are grown now, but I've never forgotten that day.

Safety at Lakes and Pools

Rising tides are not the problems at lakes and pools. All too often we read of children drowning while swimming or playing near water. Drowning is the second leading cause of death, after automobile accidents, in children up to age 14.

Watch your children constantly when they are near water, even if there is a lifeguard in attendance. Just because the pool at the campground is fenced, don't assume that everyone will close the gate behind them; a child might easily wander into the enclosure. Teach your children the buddy system, and hold buddy checks often. Don't allow them to go near water alone. Insist that they wear life vests when they are out in boats.

Check the depth of the lakes where the kids will be wading or diving. Have a good swimmer walk out to check for drop-offs or rocks on the bottom. Don't allow the kids to dive head first into water of unknown depth.

Wild Animals

When a cute chipmunk shows up at your campsite, it's hard not to want to feed the little fellow. Unfortunately, too many people were not able to resist the impulse. That's how he got the nerve to come up so close. It's important to remember that these cute little creatures are wild animals. If you feed them, you encourage them to hang around; you teach them to rely on human food, instead of foraging for themselves. If you feed it by hand, you are asking to be bitten. Wild animals could carry rabies or other diseases. If someone in your party is bitten, that person should be taken to a first-aid facility as soon as possible.

Some wild animals around campgrounds have become so conditioned to the presence of humans that they brazenly approach and invade the food supplies left out. Crows have learned to tear open garbage bags. Rodents have been known to chew through heavy nylon packs. Raccoons and bears have learned how

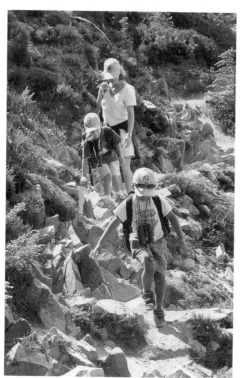
Step carefully when hiking.

to open coolers. It's not just the food that attracts these animals, it's the odors of the food. Maddy, 12, said that some very smart raccoons somehow made their way into the back of their unlocked car. Make your food supply unavailable to animals by storing food, garbage, cooking gear, and other odorous items locked in the trunk.

If that isn't possible, place all these items in a bag and hang it from a tree limb so that it is at least 16 feet from the ground and 5 feet out from the trunk. Hanging the food can be a challenge, but also a task that even young children can participate in. Carolina, 11, thought that hoisting the bucket of food up into the tree at night was her favorite part of a three-night campout.

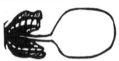

E X P E R T ' S   A D V I C E

Deterring Wildlife

If a wild animal comes into your camp, don't panic. Yelling and making as much noise as possible might frighten a bear away from your campsite. Scare off a mountain lion by making yourself look as big as possible. Raise your arms, flap your jacket overhead, and make a lot of noise.

Here's a tip: Put a rock in the toe of a sock, tie the sock to a rope, and throw it over the limb of the tree. Then attach the food bag and pull it up.

Some campgrounds have food-storage lockers in the ground or poles up in the air (like football goal posts) where you can stash your food supplies. My friend Helen called them "bruin baffles." Isaac, 12, thinks "a bear bin, which locks your food in a bucket, works better" than hanging. Eleven-year-old Clare's family had been warned by the ranger about the bears, and they saw huge metal boxes for food storage at every campsite. Nonetheless, they thought they could leave their dinner for just a moment while they went off to brush their teeth. When they came back, two bears were visiting their campsite! They yelled and made as much noise as they could, as the ranger had instructed them, and the bears ran off.

A bear once came into my campsite on the ocean at Olympic National Park while I was cooking dinner. I banged some pots together and yelled as loudly as I could. The bear left slowly.

If you are camping in bear country, make sure that no one in your party goes to bed with gum or a candy wrapper in a pocket. Don't sleep in the same clothing that you wore for cooking. Follow the 100 yard rule: Locate your food storage area 100 yards downwind from your tent. For more information about bears, go to the website for Insight Wildlife Management, www.insightwildlife.com, for a pamphlet on bears. Chris Morgan, the director, is out in the field too much to be reached by phone, but you can write to him at PO Box 28656, Bellingham, Washington 98228. Insight Wildlife seeks to nurture the role of humans as wildlife stewards through informed science and education.

In recent years, more reports have come out about mountain lion attacks. Mountain lions, also known as cougars, pumas, and wildcats, are usually quite shy. When they hunt, they look for small prey. Children are especially attractive for the cat that is ready to attack humans. If a mountain lion approaches, scare it off by raising your arms, making yourself look as big as you can, and making a lot of noise.

There are things you can do to keep predators away. When I hike, I always have a bell attached to my pack. At Banff National Park in Canada, I saw a little boy with a bell pinned to the back of his overalls, to ward off animals and

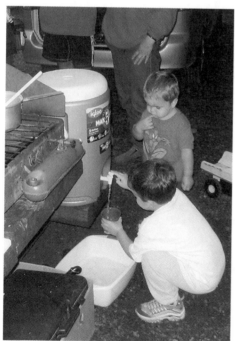

To prevent visits from critters, keep the kitchen area clean and clean up after all meals.

also so his parents could keep track of him. When Randy, his wife, and their young daughter backpack, they carry pepper spray to forestall attacks, and they make sure that their daughter, 6, walks in between her parents.

On the other hand, don't show so much concern about wild animals approaching that your children end up unnecessarily frightened. Cassandra, 11, and her friends were so scared by something "glowing" in a tree, they all rushed off screaming. The next morning, they found a brown and black cat sleeping there, and returned it to its home across the lake, from which it had been missing for several days.

You can reassure young children that nothing bad will approach your tent by spraying "critter repellant" around the boundaries. This is nothing more than a spray bottle to which you have added something with a strong odor, like vinegar or bleach. I don't know if it works against critters, but it reassures the kids.

Snakes

If you know you are going into an area where there are poisonous snakes, warn your children ahead of time not to go poking around in holes or hollow logs or stumps. If you're going to turn over a rock to investigate the life beneath, choose your rock carefully. Don't select a rock that's surrounded by thick brush. If you have a long-handled walking stick, tap gently on the rock or around its base. If you hear a rattle, back off.

What Basic First Aid Do We Need to Know?

Most parents are already skilled in treating the ordinary injuries that all active children are subject to, but in a camping situation, the potential injuries are different than those of the playground. As we set off for a camping trip, none of us expects to be faced with the necessity of dealing with poison ivy, bee stings, ticks, burns, sunburn, or diarrhea, and certainly not the more serious possibilities of sprains or broken bones, but these are all problems that we might meet.

Although I consulted several different first-aid manuals, government safety regulations, and two medical doctors (a pediatrician, Barbara Cummings, and my husband, a physician specializing in rehabilitation) to review this section, the advice is all my own.

IMAGINARY CAMPING

Handling Emergencies

Think through the potential health and accident problems of your planned camping excursion. How could you prevent them? How would you handle them?

This section is not intended to frighten parents who might be thinking about trying camping. Rather, its purpose is to alert you to some possibilities. It is not feasible to cover every mishap that might occur. Once again, this is a time for imaginary camping: Think about potential health or accident problems, and then think through the steps you would take to handle them. Better still, think about preventing problems before they happen. Consider taking a basic skills first-aid course, learn CPR (cardiopulmonary resuscitation), and keep a first-aid manual with your camping necessities. I recommend three: The *American Red Cross First Aid & Safety Handbook*, *Mountaineering Medicine*, and *Backcountry First Aid and Extended Care* (see Resources, page 242, for information about ordering these books).

It should go without saying, but I'm saying it anyway: Everyone in your party should be up to date on their tetanus immunization. If anyone is on some kind of medication, be sure you carry a supply sufficient for the entire time that you will be away from home. My husband suggests that you carry a written record of prescriptions; if your supply falls overboard from your canoe or is otherwise lost, you'll be able to replace them. If your kids are bringing friends along, talk to their parents to be sure you know of any medical problems or allergies they have.

Poisonous Plants

There are two kinds of poisonous plants—those that should not be eaten and those that should not be touched. To avoid the first kind, teach your children never to put any plant, berry, or leaf that they don't know into their mouths. Youngsters who are at the stage when everything goes into their mouths need to be watched especially carefully when they are camping.

If you're too late, if the child has already eaten something that may be poisonous, look for symptoms of unusual behavior. If you suspect that the child may have ingested a poisonous plant, get him

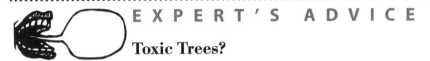

E X P E R T ' S   A D V I C E

Toxic Trees?

Remember that toxins from poisonous plants can infest clothing or shoes and migrate to other people. Even the smoke from burning those noxious plants can spread the toxins. If someone in your group has eaten a plant that you believe may be poisonous, bring a sample of the suspicious plant to the emergency room, so the attendants will know how to proceed.

or her to an emergency room as quickly as possible. Bring a sample of the suspicious plant with you, so that the attendants will know what treatment is called for.

To avoid the second kind of plant, including poison ivy, poison oak, poison sumac, nettles, and other irritating plants, educate yourself to recognize them. They will be different in different parts of the country. I found out about nettles shortly after we moved to the Northwest, when I walked through a field of knee-high green plants in shorts. We drove to a local drugstore where the pharmacist recommended that I apply Noxema. The irritation lasted only a few hours.

In many parks where the poisonous plants are endemic, there are posters with photos and knowledgeable rangers to help people watch out for them. In Seward Park in Seattle and in the Presidio in San Francisco, patches of poison oak were conveniently identified with little signs; my daughter Judy warned me not to poke my walking stick into the plants because the toxins could cling to it. Most contact poisoning is not life threatening unless the affected person has an allergy to the plant; in that case, if it's a known allergy, he or she should be carrying an antidote.

Nettles are not as dangerous as poison oak, poison ivy, and poison sumac. Redness and pain from the first disappear in a few hours. Cold compresses or soothing lotion like calamine or Noxema help the pain; so will an analgesic like Tylenol. Of course, you will use a children's compound, which you should have packed in your first-aid kit.

The effects of the other three poisons, oak, ivy, and sumac, are much more severe and last longer. Symptoms range from redness to runny blisters. Toxins from the plants can infest clothing or shoes or a walking stick and then migrate to other people. Even the smoke from burning those noxious plants can spread the toxins.

If someone in your group has the misfortune of running through a patch of one of the poisonous plants, very carefully remove their

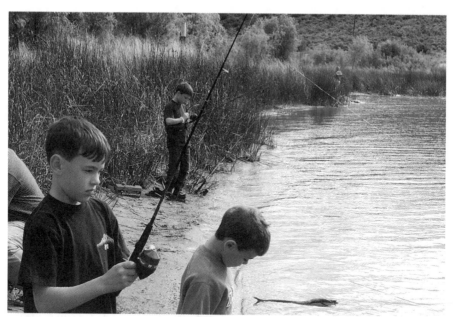

Watch out for stinging nettles and other poisonous plants on the way to your daytime activities, like fishing at a nearby lake.

clothing and put it in a bag to be laundered at home and then aired in sunlight for two days. If possible, wear latex gloves for this procedure. Wash the affected area with soap and water to keep any toxins on the skin from spreading. There is no cure for these poisons, but analgesics and soothing lotions may help. Seek medical advice if the reaction seems severe.

Bites and Stings

Avoiding bee stings and insect bites is more difficult than avoiding poisonous plants. Use bug repellent liberally to keep the little devils away, but be sure that the brand you buy is safe for children. Deet, the active ingredient in many repellents, can be absorbed through the skin, and when it is absorbed in large quantities, it can be damaging to small children. A better way to protect infants is to dress them with lightweight long-sleeved shirts and long pants.

In your first-aid kit, carry your favorite remedy to use if someone in your family is bitten or stung. Over-the-counter hydrocortisone

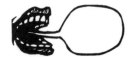

E X P E R T ' S   A D V I C E

Scent Sense

Perfumes and scented lotions may be appealing to people—but they also attract bugs! Avoid wearing perfumes or scented lotions, which will attract mosquitoes and bees to your camp.

cream is a common anti-itch treatment. Meat tenderizer, mixed with water to form a paste, will relieve a sting; it acts to denature the offending protein from the insect's sting. Again, the person who has a known allergy to bee stings should always carry an antidote.

Ticks are a variety of insect that may be new to people who have never camped. They are very small, some no bigger than the head of a pin, and they have a hard shell. Ticks bury their heads in the flesh of an animal to suck on its blood; sometimes that animal is a human or a dog. If you're visiting an area known to have ticks, like a grassy meadow, inspect your kids when you put them to bed. If you find a tick, very carefully remove it by grasping it with the tweezers from your first-aid kit and pulling slowly and steadily. Do the same thing for your dog. If the tick's bite seems inflamed, dab it with an antibiotic ointment. Wash your hands when you're done.

Insect repellants for children will help somewhat to keep ticks away. So will dressing the child in long pants and long sleeves. If you're in a known tick-infested area, tuck the child's pant legs into his or her socks.

Snake Bites

Six-year-old Sam told me the story of how he was bitten by a rattlesnake. He was throwing rocks at a bush, he said, and he didn't know that the snake was in the bush until it came out and bit him. You may wonder which isolated campground or park this happened in. It was in his grandparents' front yard in Arizona.

Sam was rushed to an emergency room, where the staff was familiar with treating snakebites. Because Sam had seen the snake, he was able to help them identify it.

Snake venom travels through the body through the lymph system, so the best help you can give someone who was bitten is to try to keep the venom from traveling. Keep that person calm and quiet while you go for help; if you have ice in your ice chest, apply it to a place that is between the bite and the heart, closer to the bite. If you choose to carry a snakebite kit in your first-aid kit, review the instructions before you leave home. Don't wait until you need to use it.

Burns

Earlier, you learned what to do if a child's clothing or hair catches fire: Stop! Drop! Roll! But what do you do when the fire is out? First, remove any smoldering clothing that is still on the child, unless it's stuck in an open wound. In that case, wait for a professional to care for it. Immerse the burn in cold water to relieve pain;

don't rub it with lotion or ointment. Cover the burn with a nonstick dressing and a loose bandage. Watch it daily for signs of infection—red streaks running away from it, swelling, or pus.

If there is broken skin or if the burn covers large areas of the body, take your burned patient to an emergency room. If the burn area is small and the skin unbroken, keep the child quiet and give him pain reliever from your first-aid kit.

Sunburn

All of us toss around the phrase SPF, but did you know that it stands for sun protection factor? We judge our sunscreens by their SPF numbers, the higher the better. My experts recommend a sunscreen with at least SPF 15; it should also be effective against both UVA and UVB rays. More important than the number, however, is the frequency with which it is applied. To be effective, sunscreen should be applied about 30 minutes before exposure, and it should be reapplied after swimming or prolonged sweating.

If, in spite of your precautions, you have a sunburned child, give him pain reliever and avoid further exposure until the discomfort is gone. That doesn't mean you need to go home; it means you

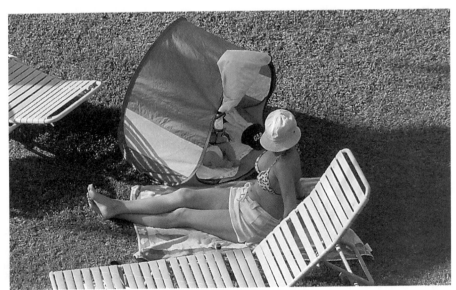

Baby is protected, but mom risks a burn. Make sure everyone wears sunscreen.

should dress the sunburned child in long pants and long sleeves, and keep him or her in the shade for a few days.

Blisters

Blisters form when skin rubs continuously against another surface, causing friction. The blisters most often found in camping situations are on the feet, and they are a direct result of poorly fitting shoes, a wrinkled sock worn on a hike, or wet socks. Some hikers wear two socks, a thin liner inside a thicker sock, but they must

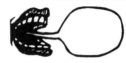

E X P E R T ' S   A D V I C E

Three Steps for Avoiding Blisters

1. Be sure your kids' shoes fit correctly.

2. Be sure that their socks are pulled on smoothly with no wrinkles.

3. If their socks get wet, change into dry socks as soon as possible.

have a shoe large enough to accommodate this bulk. If your kids have been wearing shoes with one thin or medium-thickness sock, don't try to force their feet into thick socks.

If, in spite of your care, your child develops a blister, leave it alone if it is unbroken. It will heal itself. Protect the area for the next hike by layering moleskin around but not over the blister so there is no pressure on it. Ring-shaped pads with a hole in the middle or one of the new liquid bandage products will also protect the blister if you have one of them in your first-aid kit. If the blister is broken, dab it with a little antibiotic ointment and protect it with a bandage. If the blister area becomes very red, very warm, or very painful, it may be infected; in that case, seek medical attention.

Diarrhea and Dehydration

Among your favorite remedies in your first-aid kit, you should have packed something for diarrhea. Since diarrhea is often caused by eating something contaminated or not properly stored, chances are that more than one person in the family will be affected. While you're waiting for the medication to take effect, the affected people should be encourage to drink lots of safe fluids, like plain, clean water, and to eat the BRAT diet, bananas, rice, applesauce, and toast, a combination easier for distressed intestines to digest.

If you think the diarrhea might be caused by some contaminated food, get rid of anything not properly stored for even a short time, and get extra stern about hand-washing and hand sanitizer use. If you think the water in camp may be the culprit, boil it for five minutes and then let it cool before anyone drinks it.

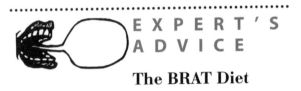

EXPERT'S ADVICE

The BRAT Diet

For diarrhea, follow the BRAT diet: Eat bananas, rice, applesauce, and toast.

When diarrhea is severe or if it has gone on for several days, you need to be concerned about dehydration. Pack rehydrating drinks, like Gatorade, or make your own from the formula SOG, which stands for sodium, orange juice, glucose. (I prefer to think of it as SOS, salt, orange juice, sugar, but those letters were taken.) Stir one-half teaspoon salt and one tablespoon sugar into a quart of orange juice; try to get your child to drink one ounce for each pound of body weight over a period of four hours. In other words, a 30-pound child would have to drink almost a quart (32 ounces) or approximately one cup per hour.

If it's possible, check the child's urine. Urine should not be dark; that is a bad sign. It should be the color of straw.

Vomiting

Another cause of dehydration is vomiting. The BRAT diet will probably not work for a child who is continuously vomiting. Try to get the sick child to take some liquids. Some parents find that the only liquid that stays down is a 7-Up-type soft drink, stirred a little to take some of the carbonation out. If a child is continuously vomiting and has a fever, it's probably a good idea to go home and contact your healthcare provider.

Foreign Body in the Eye

Your first-aid kit should contain over-the-counter eye drops that can be used to flush the eye. If you don't have eye drops, use clean water.

Problems from Heat, Problems with Cold

If the temperature goes up or down, it can affect your children's health. Avoid extreme physical activity when it is very hot. This is a time for the quiet games you brought along. Stay in the shade, dress lightly, and drink lots of fluids. Heat can rise very rapidly in a parked camper; even a tent can become almost unbearable. Watch for signs of heat exposure—excessive sweating, headache, and muscle cramps. If you see these signs in your children, cool them off with wet cloths and give them fluids.

When young campers get cold and wet, parents should be watchful for signs of hypothermia, which is low body temperature brought on

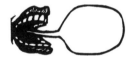

E X P E R T ' S   A D V I C E

Not Too Hot, Not Too Cold

To help keep warm or cool, fluids are important: Give cool drinks when the children are too hot and warm drinks when they are too cold.

by chilling. Symptoms include shivering, slurred speech, unsteady gait, and irrational behavior. Hypothermia is treated by warming; give warm fluids and put the child in a heated bed or in a sleeping bag with another person to provide body warmth. Hypothermia is prevented by keeping the children warm and dry, with proper rain gear and hats. If you're caught away from camp, waiting out a downpour, try to stay out of the wind. If the kids get soaked, get them into warm and dry clothing as soon as possible.

Be especially watchful of infants in carriers on cold, windy days, even if it isn't raining. Children in carriers are not generating heat through exercise; they need extra layers of clothing and windproof outer layers to stay warm. Check them often for signs of chilling. Feel their arms or legs, and watch for shivering.

Broken Bones, Sprains, and Strains

A few years ago, I broke three bones in my leg in a classic skiing accident, a slow, twisting fall where my binding didn't release. As soon as the offending binding was removed, the pain lessened considerably. I thought I had probably sprained my ankle, but I had the good sense not to try to get up and ski down on it. I sat up and packed snow around my boot. When the ski patrol arrived, they took me down in a toboggan. I didn't realize there were broken bones until the x-ray tech in the emergency room told me so.

> ### Quick Quiz
>
> #### Safety in Numbers
>
> **Q:** How many people do you need to treat an injury?
>
> **A:** Three. One to tend the injured, one to go for help, and one to watch over the other children.

When a bone or a joint has been twisted or injured, there is no way to tell if it is a sprain, a muscle strain, or a fracture until it is x-rayed. Don't try to pre-guess the professionals. You can do a lot of harm by trying to use a broken bone.

If you think the injury might be a broken bone in an arm or a leg, immobilize the limb with some kind of splint. When my leg was broken, the ski patrolmen put it in a corrugated cardboard box and put plastic bags filled with snow around it. If you have a box, cut it down to fit the limb, and use all the ice in your ice chest to fill plastic bags. If you don't have a box, create a makeshift splint from something stiff that is the right length; my nephew wrapped a foam pad around his friend's broken leg. Put the arm or leg on a pillow with the splint and gently tie them together with a sweater or a shirt. If a broken bone is sticking out of the flesh, don't try to put it back; keep the injured limb as still as possible.

An Injured Person

In the event of an injury, call for medical help immediately. If the campground you are staying at has a manager, a ranger, or a host, inform that person. They will know the fastest way to get help. If you're in a campground that is not attended and someone in the camp has a working cell phone, call 911 for instructions.

But what if you are in an isolated campground and the phone doesn't work? Ideally, in this emergency situation, there would be

••

Three Good Books on First Aid

1. *Backcountry First Aid and Extended Care* by Buck Tilton (Falcon 2002)
2. *Mountaineering Medicine* by Fred T. Darvill, Jr. M.D. (Wilderness Press 1998)
3. *American Red Cross First Aid & Safety Handbook* by Kathleen A. Handal (Little Brown 1992)

••

three responsible adults: one to tend the injured, one to go for help, and one to watch over the other children. But in a less than ideal situation, someone will have to make the decision: who stays, who goes?

When you're camping, the closest 911 facility may be miles and miles away. A family may decide to bring the injured person to the emergency room rather than wait for emergency medical technicians to arrive in camp. That's why you should know where the hospital nearest your campground is located.

Don't try to move the injured person if you think there might be a neck or spinal injury. Ambulance technicians carry special collars and back boards for moving people with such injuries. You can do a lot of harm by trying to move that person yourself.

If the injured person is bleeding, apply pressure to the wound with a cloth of some kind for at least five minutes. Continue the pressure; don't peek to see if the bleeding has stopped. Don't try to sterilize the wound.

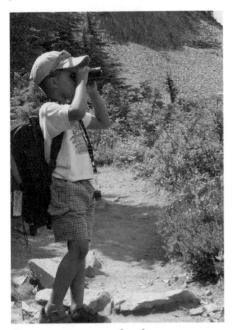

Keep an eye on each other so no one gets lost.

A friend sent me an article by Mark Oberle, M.D., M.P.H., of the University of Washington, who happened to be vacationing in Thailand during the 2004 tsunamis. Dr. Oberle wrote, "...the only real first-aid priority is to stop bleeding, primarily through direct pressure... with gauze or bandages or any sort of cloth..." He goes on to say that if the wound will not be attended to for a day or more, it should be cleaned with plain water. "There is no benefit from antiseptic (especially one like alcohol) at this stage. Soap and water, possibly OK...but the main need is to remove debris, not sterilization. Something painful, like alcohol, would probably not cause much damage, but would cause unnecessary pain, with no real benefit."

If removal to the emergency room is your decision, move your vehicle as close to the injured person as you can get it. Get some help lifting, if possible, so that the injured person is jostled as little as possible during the move.

Although this is an emergency, don't create more problems by a hasty departure. Your campfire should be completely out. Everyone in the car should be safely belted in. As you get closer to the hospital, have someone in the vehicle keep testing your cell phone. When it works, telephone ahead to 911 so that they know you're on your way.

What if Someone is Lost?

Getting lost is one of the most frightening of camp accidents, for both parents and children. It can happen very easily. This is another misadventure easier to prevent than to remedy.

Some years ago, my daughter and I left the cabin where we were staying high above the ocean, walked down a path through a densely wooded ravine, and took a walk on the beach. When it was time to head back, we couldn't find the path; there was no break in the dense woods. We walked miles before we came to a cliff we could scale, climbed over a fence, and walked back along the road. My husband said he knew where we were going because he could follow the distinctive patterns of our shoes. The family was distraught. We could have avoided the commotion if we had stopped to tie a piece of bright tape to the woods when we came out on the beach.

Ali, 12, wrote about a family history that her mother had passed down to her. When the mother was a child, her parents and four children had stopped for lunch at a rest stop, and one son, 9, wandered off. After lunch, three kids hopped in the car and the parents drove off. Ali said, "After traveling a while in silence, everyone in the car realized they were short one person!" They quickly turned back and found the boy waiting calmly at the table where they had eaten. Weren't they lucky? They found their boy, and he had confidence that his family would come back and find him.

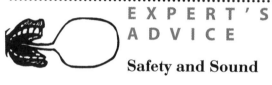

EXPERT'S ADVICE

Safety and Sound

Develop a signal for your family whistle, so you can find each other if you get separated in camp or on the trail.

The child who wanders away for 15 minutes may not show that he has been harmed, but the psychological aftereffects for child and parent could linger a long, long time. Make sure that your children understand the boundaries of your campsite. If you have a toddler who loves to wander, one adult should take responsibility for that child, setting aside for a time other camp tasks.

Older, more responsible children should have a whistle with them at all times, and parents should have a whistle, too. Develop a signal so that you can find each other: two shorts, one long, for example. Don't put the whistle on a string around the child's neck; he or she could be strangled if the cord caught on a bush or a tree. Put the whistle on a cord long enough to reach from the child's pocket to his mouth, pin the end to the pocket, and stuff all inside.

If a child, even an older one capable of managing for himself, leaves the trail on a hike to go into the woods to pee or poop, an adult should go along and wait a discreet but short distance away. It's easy to become disoriented in a deep forest and lose the way back.

Give each of your children who are old enough to go off by themselves some pieces of brightly colored trail-marking tape. Carry some yourself. Use it to mark the fork in the trail that you take, or the wooded entrance to the trail. Teach your children to look back often. The return trail looks different from the outbound trail. It's easy to miss a turnoff if you haven't marked it. On the way back, the last person should be sure to untie the tape and bring it back. You can use it again, and it won't litter the environment. If you don't have tape, draw an arrow in the dirt with your heel or a stick, or make an arrow out of little stones. Scatter the arrow on your way back.

Five Basic Things To Tell Your Kids If They Get Lost

1. I will not be angry at you.
2. I will get lots of people to help look for you.
3. Sit down and stay there and wait for me.
4. Wrap up in something warm.
5. Don't be afraid to talk to strangers in this situation.

If your child is going to leave your campsite by himself or with others, make sure you know where they plan to go, just as you have told someone at home, a relative or a neighbor, where you have gone. A child who is technologically adept could have a walkie-talkie. We see many of them in campgrounds.

A younger child could be outfitted with the Angel Alert. This small, two-part transmitter/receiver (one for the parent and one attached to the child) operates on a lithium battery. It's an early-warning system that detects when the child strays too far from adult supervision. The transmitter has a panic button, so a child can radio a parent when he or she has gone too far. I saw it at Portland Luggage; you can find out more at www.angelalert.net.

Some people carry a little survival kit. You and your children could make one together. Find a little metal box with a tight-fitting, hinged lid; this is a task by itself. Mine is an old Band-Aid box, from the days when Band-Aids came in a metal box. A mint or a tea container might work. If you can't find a box, use a small Ziploc bag. The container should be kept in the child's backpack, if he or

HELPING HANDS

Survival Kit

You and your child can made a survival kit containing a waterproof wrap, a whistle, and some hard candy to be used only in an emergency.

she carries one; otherwise, it should be small enough to fit in the child's jacket pocket.

Put into your container something wind-and-waterproof to wrap up in, like a Mylar rescue blanket or a plastic trash bag that has been slit for a face. Help your child roll up the bag and press all the air out, so it scrunches into a tiny packet. Add a whistle. If you wish, put in a package of Life Savers or other long-lasting candy. Teach your child that these items are to be used only in an emergency. Show your child how the slit in the trash bag allows his or her face to peek out.

"Hug-A-Tree and Survive" and "Stay Put, Stay Dry"

There are two organizations that I know of, one on each coast, that are dedicated to teaching children what to do if they become lost. Both Hug-A-Tree and Survive and Stay Put, Stay Dry put on programs to teach children and their parents, first, what to do to stay found, and then what to do if they are lost. Both recommend that children who think they are lost should be told to pick a tree or a rock and stay with it. Both recommend that children carry a whistle and some kind of waterproof wrap, like a plastic trash bag.

(Again, teach the children to tear a hole in the top of the bag for their face, so when they put it over their heads, they won't suffocate.)

Teach your children that if they are lost, the worst thing to do is to start running. Children who think they are lost tend to get panicky and start running around; then they get hot so they peel off and lose their clothing; then they get chilled. Tell your children not to take off their jackets or their hats even if they feel hot. Tell them to sit down and wait for someone to find them.

Promise your children that you will not be angry at them for getting lost. Some kids believe that their parents will be mad at them; some say their parents would never spend a lot of money to have lots of people look for them. Assure them that you will get a lot of help to find them and that it is OK in this situation to talk to strangers. Let them know that they have lots of caring people who will be looking for them. If they hear strange yelling, they should yell back. If it's an animal, it will be frightened away, but more likely it will be a searcher, who will find them and return them to their parents.

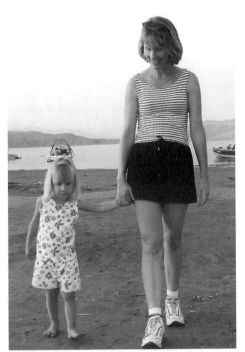

Going on a walk? Bring a buddy!

Hug-A-Tree adds, make yourself big and visible; show your brightest colors, and if a plane flies overhead, lie down in a clear space. A person lying down is bigger and easier to spot from the air than a person standing up.

The Philadelphia Hug-A-Tree program had several suggestions for parents: They suggest "footprinting" your child by spreading a piece of aluminum foil on a soft surface, like a carpet or a folded towel, and having the child walk across it. Mark the foil with the child's name. (This assumes that your child will be wearing his or her hiking shoes for the footprint.) This record will enable trackers to separate your child's prints from others in the area, and determine the direction of search much more quickly. They also say that parents should call for search and rescue quickly, if they think their child is lost. One more way that parents can assist in the search is to be available in the search area; often clues from family and friends lead to finding a child in good shape.

Stay Put, Stay Dry adds these precautions: Hike in a group or with a buddy; count the number of people you start out with and keep track of them; tell someone where you are going and when you will return; don't eat or drink anything you didn't bring with you. As its name suggests, this organization emphasizes staying warm by staying dry.

Hug-a-Tree and Survive was started in San Diego, California, in 1981, after 9-year-old Jimmy Beveridge died of exposure about 2 miles from his campground. The program, dedicated to Jimmy, has been picked up by sheriffs' offices and search and rescue organizations all over the US and Canada. If they have a program in your area, they will put on a presentation for your organization. To find out if they have program near you, call the Hug-a-Tree main office at 619-286-7536 or visit their website for more information: www.sdsheriff.net/SAR/pr/hugatree.html.

Stay Put, Stay Dry was started by Eastern Mountain Sports (EMS) in 2004 after a 10-year-old boy died of exposure in New Hampshire. EMS is a retailer with more than 80 retail stores across 16 states. EMS also teaches climbing and mountaineering classes. Their free Stay Put, Stay Dry program is offered in all their stores as a public service biannually. For more information, go to their website, www.ems.com, and click on Store Locator. Find the store nearest your home and contact the store manager to see when the program will be offered.

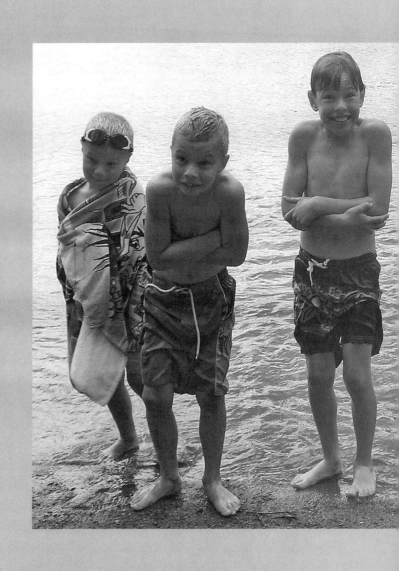

Beyond Camping
Leaving the Car Behind

▶ River Rafting

▶ Boating

▶ Horse-Supported
Camping or Riding

▶ Backpacking

▶ Canoeing

▶ Bicycle Touring

When our older two children reached teen years, they grew less interested in camping as a family. My daughter said she was tired of all the green forests in the Northwest, but they agreed to take one last big family trip, hiking in the red hills of Utah. As a treat, I signed us up for an overnight rafting trip on the Colorado River. The teens were unhappy with the idea; they said they would be bored sitting around on a boat all day.

As it turned out, it was a very exciting trip. The teens chose to ride in another boat, without parents, so we had only the youngest with us. When there were no rapids, the guides allowed passengers to jump in, wearing life vests, and float down the river. We slept in tents on the bank and ate great meals that the crew prepared over a fire. It was there I first saw Dutch oven cooking. At the end, when the teens saw that the river went on while we were disembarking, they were unhappy that I had signed on for such a short trip.

Once your family has tried and enjoyed camping, there are numerous other outdoor adventures in which you can apply the skills you learned as campers: river rafting, boating, houseboating, horse-supported hiking, riding trips, canoeing, or bike touring.

River Rafting

No one should get bored on a whitewater rafting trip. If you go with a rafting company, it is a combination of luxurious camping with a thrilling, Disneyland-type ride, except that it lasts a lot longer. It's a wonderful family activity, but not for families with infants or toddlers. All rafting companies have an age limit and some have a height limit as well. But once you qualify, prepare for the time of your life. If you are an expert rafter and you take your own family, it becomes more work; then it is like backpacking on water.

Rafting with an outfitter is the easiest of camping trips. All companies provide all the food and the cooks for all meals, in order to avoid any food contamination. Food poisoning on the river would be a dreadful situation. You may be shocked, as I was, at the amount of food that is thrown away, but once it has been removed from the cooler and served, it can't be served again.

Depending on the company a family contracts with, the rafters may also supply tents, sleeping bags, and dry bags, or they may ask you to provide your own. Dry bags are heavy waterproof bags that allow your clothing and personal items to travel through giant waves without getting wet. If you're doing your own trip, you have to organize all this equipment, plus rafts and food.

A rafting trip usually begins with a demonstration of packing and rolling the dry bag. When they're going to be wet most of the time, rafters really need only one extra set of clothing, something dry to put on at the end of the day. The limiting dry bag forces you to leave a lot behind, and the company usually has some means of storing your extra clothing. Nylon shorts and a T-shirt, or a two-piece swimsuit with a light-weight shirt over it, is fine for the girls; shorts and a shirt work for the boys. If it rains, you'll need a light-weight rain suit; on one of our trips, the company supplied these.

CHECKLIST

River Health and Safety

▶ Follow boatmen's instructions for pee and poop.

▶ Carry all waste out properly.

▶ Plan sufficiently so that you don't keep meats or cooked foods over from one meal to the next.

▶ Drink lots of fluids.

▶ Wear a life jacket on the river at all times.

Everyone should be wearing lots of sunscreen and reapplying it often. If the boatmen don't supply a sturdy "ammo" box or a mesh bag that ties onto the boat to keep the sunscreen handy, you should bring your own. All should wear hats that tie on, and sunglasses, which also should be strapped on. You're going on a wild ride!

The boatmen will give you a lecture on river hygiene. Depending on the trip, if you are rafting through a very dry area, you will be told to pee in the river or on wet sand; the portable potties that the boats carry are for poop only. You may be told to burn your toilet paper in a tin can that will be cached, with matches, near the potty. Do this very carefully; a few years ago, some Harvard students in the North Cascades tried to burn their toilet paper and set a fire that burned thousands of acres.

You will also be instructed on how to dispose of waste after meals and how to wash your dishes. Many companies expect you to keep your own dishes separate as a hygienic measure. Some ask you to provide your own unbreakable dishes, with a mesh bag to keep them in.

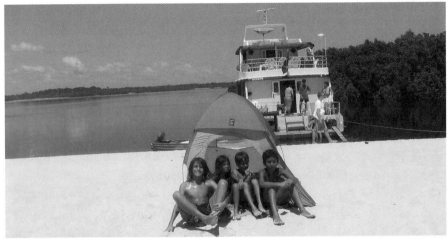

On this boat trip, the kids tent on the beach while the parents sleep on board.

Some companies tell you to bring a lot of canned water, soda, or beer, because you lose a lot of fluid out in the sun. These companies also provide water and often lemonade, in big coolers. It's important to drink a lot, and especially watch your children to see that they drink a lot and frequently. In my experience, there are always more cans of drinks than we could possibly consume, but it makes for some lively shake-and-spray battles between rafts.

I have been impressed with the safety measures of the boatmen with whom I have traveled. We were always instructed carefully on how we were to proceed through the rapids. The children were told to wear their life vests at all times in the boats and when they were playing at the edge of the river during time on land. Of the many different kinds of rafts, my preference is for paddle rafts that hold six or eight, with larger rafts carrying our gear, but I have also taken trips where twelve guests and two crew rode in motorized rafts with a pile of gear under a tarp in the middle. My youngest son was 11 when we took our first trip, in big four-tube inflatable J-boats. We sat on a wooden seat that spanned the boat and held on tight.

You can find rafting companies on the internet. Most companies conduct trips on more than one river. Talk to them about which trips would be most suitable for your family.

Boating

When I told Sandy and Chuck I was writing this book, she said she would never need to be an RV camper. She told me their boat is their RV. As she described their boating adventures, it sounded very much like an RV vacation. Depending on the size of the boat, it can be compared to a motorhome or to a truck camper. Preparations are the same, including packing, planning the meals, and getting the boat ready. Their boat has a refrigerator, small freezer, and stove. Just as the furnishings in an RV can be folded out or down to create sleeping space, so in the boat does the table and settee fold out of the way. Just as items in the RV must be stowed for travel, so all loose items in the boat must be "battened down" (that's sailors' talk) while they are underway.

CHECKLIST

Overnight Boating

▶ How much fuel do we have?

▶ How much fresh water do we have?

▶ How much food do we have?

▶ Where can we acquire all of the above on our trip?

Like other campers, vacationing boaters may sail from one port to another every day, staying at marinas or anchoring in quiet coves at night. The Puget Sound has state and provincial parks that are accessible only by boat. Boaters can make reservations to stay at marinas, or they can cruise in, hoping to find a spot. Sometimes they stay for more than one night, enjoying the area where they are docked. Boaters use books of charts, available at boating stores, which include maps of waterways and also list marinas and sources for food, fuel, and water.

Sandy told me about cruising into isolated coves where there were "mooring pots," buoys with a loop on the top where boats can tie a line. Tying to a buoy is safer than anchoring, she said, because anchors may drift if a wind comes up during the night. Sandy said her husband sleeps better tied to a mooring pot than when they are at anchor.

Not all boats are as large as RVs. Some boats not fitted with bunks for overnight are still found in isolated coves, but these boaters are like tent campers. They tie up to a dock and bring their tents, stoves, coolers and other camping equipment on to the shore and spend the night on land. Other boaters may continue to travel through the night with one person always awake and at the helm.

Just as RVs can be rented, so can boats. Both saltwater and freshwater rentals are available. Look to the internet and/or the yellow pages to find rental agencies in the area you are interested in, or visit a boat show to see what is available.

Boaters, like RV campers, must monitor their supplies of fuel and water carefully. Sandy said that freshwater is particularly critical, because some stops that sell fuel do not have fresh water.

Freshwater is necessary for rinsing off when they you cruising in saltwater, Sandy said, because it is imperative that no one bring saltwater into the interior of the boat. If someone tracked salt onto the carpet, or sat on an upholstered seat while wearing a salt-soaked swimsuit, the salt would never dry out. It would absorb moisture from the air, leading to dampness and mold.

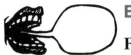

E X P E R T ' S   A D V I C E
Renting a Boat

Ask a lot of questions when you rent the boat: How old is it, when and how was it last serviced, what problems did previous renters have? Ask them for names of previous renters whom you might contact for recommendations for the company. If the renting company asks you a lot of questions about your plans, don't be annoyed; they are probably more conscientious about caring for their boats than other companies that don't ask questions.

If the children swim or wade in saltwater, they have to be doused with freshwater before they can come back into the cabin. Sandy keeps "sun showers" on deck for that purpose, and special saltwater towels that don't get co-mingled with the rest of the laundry. Sun showers are heavy plastic water bags, black on one side, that sit out in the sun and absorb heat. The swimsuits are kept out of the cabin.

Sandy and Chuck both agreed vehemently that the most important rule for boating with children is that the kids must always wear life vests when they are on the deck, where there are open railings, or on the dock. There are no exceptions. When they are underway and the children are down in the cabin, they can remove the vests, but the vests are kept right next to the entry to be donned when the kids come up.

On one of their trips, when they had a toddler along, they fastened a D-ring to her life vest, and put a line through it that was tied to the railing at each side of the deck. She could move back and forth along the line, but she could not fall out of the boat.

Like other campers, the children enjoy finding other children to play with in marinas and on shore, but on the docks all the kids are expected to wear life vests. While they are underway, Sandy's kids play board or card games, read, or do art projects. Sometimes they fish from the dock, or from the dinghy that trails behind the bigger boat. Some families have TV sets and DVDs on board, but Sandy won't allow them. If only one of their children is with them, they take a friend along so she will have company.

Houseboating

After years of camping together and watching their children grow older, Ricki and Michael's group decided to try something different—houseboating. Seven families—36 people—arranged to rent two house boats on a lake in Canada. There were 18 on each boat. A year later, a smaller group went to a different rental marina to rent one house boat.

These boats, they said, were like trailers on pontoons. Each had a full kitchen, a generator for a TV and a VCR, and an electrically operated toilet. In addition to the houseboats, the group rented two jet skis, which they all took turns riding, and they brought along inner tubes and an inflatable raft.

While they were out on the skis or the tubes, everyone wore a life vest, but since all their children were older and good swimmers, they didn't insist on the vests on the boat. The jet skis made all the difference to the teenagers among them, who would otherwise have been bored with the slow pace.

Houseboating is much like cruising, except that houseboaters do not cover the same longer distances. The group drove up to the marina, unloaded their food and other gear, and, after a bit of instruction, set out. The two boats traveled separately, but they met at an agreed-upon beach each evening. Each group did their own shopping, meal planning, and cooking. At night, they spread their sleeping bags on the fold-down bunks inside or on the deck outside. The children moved back and forth, sleeping on one boat one night, the other another.

Problems arose on one trip when the electrically operated toilet wouldn't work while the boat was underway, so whoever needed to flush had to call out to the boat driver to cut the engine.

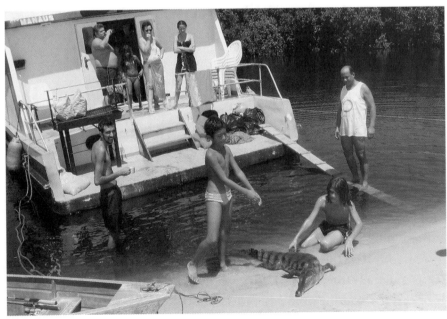

On a boat, you may encounter exotic wildlife.

At night the houseboats didn't need a dock or a marina. They pulled up close to the beach and tied two lines, one from each side of the square front of the boat, to a tree or to a stake driven into the ground. Wind could have been a problem. The big square boats caught the wind like a sail and the boats could have been turned sideways into the shore, where it would have been difficult to get them away.

Michael told me there was a big difference between the two rental companies. The first they found through the internet; the second was a neighboring business they noted on the first trip. One company asked a lot of questions before they rented: Who was renting, what their experience had been, how many people, and so on. The other company was more lackadaisical, Michael said, and just agreed to the rental. But the first company's boats were in much better condition than the second; although the questioning had been annoying, it turned out that their boats were better taken care of.

In retrospect, the group agreed that tent camping was easier to organize than houseboating, and one boat had been easier to manage than two. Food became an issue when the large group shopped and shared dinners.

Horse-Supported Camping or Riding

If you're a mountain family rather than a river or lake family, you're not excluded from luxury camping. There are companies that will take you into the mountains for a span of days, traveling either on foot or on horseback, from one beautiful campsite to another. They may provide all the food and a cook, or they may expect you to provide the food and cook it yourself. The luxury comes from the horse, or, with some companies, a llama. If you're riding, the horse is doing all the work. If you're hiking, a pack animal carries all your heavy gear and you carry only a daypack with your lunch, rain gear, and perhaps a camera.

EXPERT'S ADVICE
Luxury and Adventure

If you're ready for adventure but not a lot of work, consider my favorite form of luxury camping: horse-supported camping. When a pack animal carries all my heavy gear, I need carry only a daypack with my lunch, rain gear, and a camera.

My favorite such company is run by the Ray Courtney family, which operates Cascade Corrals out of Stehekin, Washington, an isolated settlement at the head of Lake Chelan. It can be reached only by boat, hiking trail, or float plane. Cascade Corrals butts up against the boundary of North Cascades National Park, but there are other companies in other mountains that offer similar services

The Courtney family runs strings of horses. When you sign up for a hiking or trail-riding vacation, they send you a duffel bag that you must use for all of your gear, including your sleeping bag. A horse

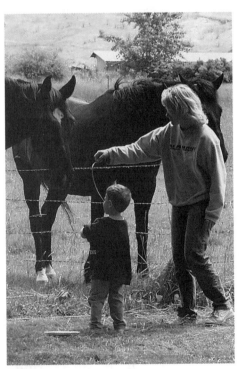

Tired of hiking? Let a horse take you camping.

will carry it, and also your tent, which they provide. They also supply a wrangler for the horses, a cook, and all your food.

The Courtneys have an age limit of 12 for children, but they say they can make exceptions when one family contracts for the whole trip. They can also schedule a private trip for a minimum of 12 hikers or six riders. I've been on Courtney trips with hiking children aged 8 or 9 who had no trouble keeping up with the rest of us. I've also seen kids younger than 12 riding their horses. A private trip can be tailored to the limits you know your kids can handle. The Cascade Corrals website is www.courtneycountry.com. You can write to them at PO Box 67, Stehekin, Washington 98852.

You can also find companies that will send you out with one or two burros or llamas. Small children can ride on the burro, so that may be a better choice for young families. If you have a wrangler going with you to be responsible for the animals, you are more free to enjoy the scenery and your family, but you have less privacy. On the other hand, you may not wish to take responsibility for somebody else's llama.

There are lots of ways to find these companies. Use the internet, or, if you know the area you'd like to visit, use the state tourism information services to find out what is available. Ask a lot of questions, especially about their experience with children, and be sure to find out what the company provides and what they expect of you.

Backpacking

I wrote a whole book called *Backpacking with Babies and Small Children*, also based on interviewing a lot of people, so it's hard to condense all that information into the few paragraphs here.

Backpacking is an exercise in responsibility. When you backpack, you must carry everything that you need for the night or two that you will be out. If you backpack with your children, you may end up carrying everything that the children need, and possibly the children themselves. Backpackers also must be prepared to handle

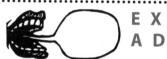

E X P E R T ' S A D V I C E

Your First Time in the Backcountry

First backpacking trips with the kids should be no more than 2 or 3 miles from the trailhead.

any emergency, change of weather, or injury. It's not like camping in a campground, where you can jump into your car and drive to the nearest town.

If you're contemplating moving on from car camping to back-packing, practice imaginary camping again. Look at your camping equipment. Ask yourself how many cooking pots you really need. How many changes of clothing? Look at your menu and consider how many ounces each item weighs.

How much each person can carry depends on the fitness of that person, the distance you will travel, and the elevation gain to the

IMAGINARY CAMPING

Backpacking

Look at your camping equipment and think about what you don't really need, especially if you're the one who's going to carry it. Think about the weight of the child you may also be carrying, or the weight of the child's pack if one of the kids decides he or she can't carry it anymore.

next stop. Test your family's abilities by taking long walks in the neighborhood wearing packs that weigh approximately the same as the ones they will wear on the backpack trip. At the same time, you can check to see that the packs are comfortable.

Successful backpackers have lists of the absolute necessities that they must have with them, but they've also learned what they can leave behind. It's not the same for everyone. In my family, each of us is allowed one large plastic cup and one spoon. At breakfast, we choose whether to have oatmeal that tastes like cocoa, or cocoa that tastes like oatmeal, because we each have only one cup.

We carry a lightweight single-burner stove and a teakettle for boiling water; that's the extent of our kitchen. All of our dinners are freeze-dried meals that can be reconstituted in their bags and eaten from the cups. If we buy dried soups in Styrofoam cups, we re-pack them at home in small Ziploc bags. Lunches consist of Melba toast rounds with something to spread on them and dried fruit. When the kids were little, they called the raisins and apricot halves "dried eyes and ears." Compare that to the elaborate breakfasts and the foil-wrapped or multicourse dinners of the campers next to their RVs.

As soon as our children were old enough to have a small pack, we tried to encourage them to carry some of their own things. They all had rain gear; rain gear is not something you can leave behind, even when the sun is shining and the sky is clear. They had warm layers to wear at night and one set of long underwear to sleep in, but otherwise we all wore the same outfits every day. We stashed some clean shirts in the car, so we could present a clean front if we stopped on the way home for an ice-cream cone.

CHECKLIST

Ten Essentials for Backpacking

1. Extra clothing—be prepared to layer
2. Extra food—come home with a little left over
3. Sunglasses for all
4. Knife—each adult should have one
5. Fire starter—we carry old candle stubs
6. First-aid kit
7. Matches in a waterproof container
8. Flashlight with extra bulb and batteries
9. Map
10. Compass

As the children grew older, we encouraged them to carry some of the family's food and also some lightweight piece of our common equipment, like the teakettle or the water filter or the extra canister of propane. If they had so wished, they could have brought toys, but experience taught them that toys were weighty objects best left behind.

My husband and I carried the major portion of our goods. I remember carrying two sleeping bags and a small tent, while my husband carried three sleeping bags and the other tent. He always carried a large first-aid kit, and we both carried lots of water, which is heavy. For safety's sake, we always carry the famous Ten Essentials. We never build fires; the matches and fire starter are for emergencies.

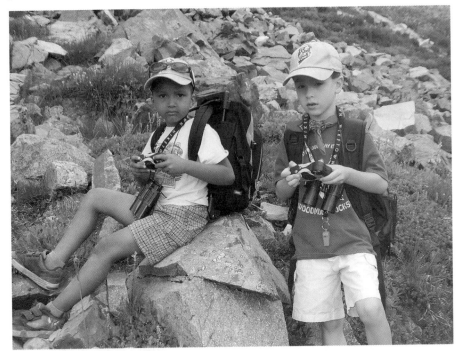

These kids are able to carry some of the family gear.

All of our children were able to walk by themselves when we began backpacking. For the backpacking book, I talked to a couple with twin infants; each parent carried one baby and half the family's equipment. I also talked to parents who enlisted a third person, or a fourth, a willing grandparent or two, who took some of the general load in addition to their own.

I talked to families who had developed creative solutions to taking their kids along. Some parents split their responsibilities by having one person walk slowly with the kids, while the other made two round trips between car and campsite, transporting heavy loads. We met a mother with four children huddled together under a tree by the side of the trail, while their father went back and forth, up and down, collecting the packs that the kids had abandoned along the way.

Our first trips were not lengthy. We tried to find destinations that were no more than 2 or 3 miles from the trailhead—hardly remote wilderness, but if we were lucky, no one else would arrive at that remote lake or river. That wasn't always possible; some parks are so popular that camping permits are required, even in the backcountry, and the backcountry camps would have more than one campsite.

You may be asking, Why bother? What does backpacking have that camping next to the car doesn't have? I think it is the sense of accomplishment that backpacking brings that is so satisfying. When I reach a mountain lake under my own steam, I know that I

HELPING HANDS
Sharing the Load

Encourage the children to carry some of the family's food and also some lightweight piece of common equipment.

have earned the right through my own hard work to see this almost pristine lake, and that no one else can see it unless they, too, are willing to put out the effort that it took to get here. I like the thought that I can be content with a minimum amount of goods, without the elaborate kitchen and the comfortable house. I hope my children are learning that happiness doesn't come from owning a lot of things.

Canoeing

While canoe camping is not an activity for infants or toddlers, it is fine for children who are strong swimmers and are old enough to take direction readily.

Like backpacking, canoe camping is an activity that requires thoughtful and thorough preparation. Everything you need for your overnight must be carried in your craft. Read the section on backpacking for ideas on what you need. You can probably take more elaborate meals and more goods with you in the canoe than in a backpack, but everything must be carefully wrapped to keep water out, and your vessel must be carefully loaded so that your gear won't unbalance it.

Parents who are thinking about taking their children on a canoe camping trip should already be skilled at operating a canoe. If both parents are experienced paddlers, they may want to take two canoes instead of one large one, which gives the family even more room to store food and changes of clothing.

The overnight camping trip should not be the children's first canoeing experience. They should have had ample opportunity to become comfortable with the canoe, to learn how to get into it and out of it quickly and safely, and to have had more than one experience with swamping it, righting it, and climbing back into it. Start with short day trips on small, sheltered lakes before you begin anything major, and remember that it's always more scenic and safe to paddle around the shores of a lake than to cross over the middle.

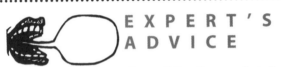

EXPERT'S ADVICE

Capable Canoeists?

For a family canoe camping trip, you need parents and children who are strong swimmers already skilled at canoeing.

For a longer trip, follow a route outlined in a canoeing guide book for that area, or use a canoeing map or a topographical map published by the US Geological Survey. Keep your map handy but secure. If it isn't waterproof, put it in a plastic bag and tuck it under a cord or tape it with duct tape in front of you. Don't let the wind catch your map and blow it away. Route finding can be tricky on the water. Some areas have designated water "trails," but the markers are often far apart.

Everyone on the canoe trip should wear a properly fitting life vest at all times. They should also wear warm clothing that will dry quickly. The new lightweight fabrics work well, with a light wind and waterproof layer over them.

Canoeing can be misleading. The canoe sits right in the water, where the temperature of the water is often much lower than the temperature of the air. One resource recommends the 120° rule: Carry a thermometer and check the temperature of the air every

CHECKLIST

Pocket Survival Kit

► Matches in a waterproof container

► A signaling mirror

► Whistle

► Space blanket

► Second copy of your map

► Compass

► Canoe repair kit

morning; then check the temperature of the water when you put in. When the combined temperatures add up to 120°F or more, the kids can begin to shed layers.

Although most of your gear will be packed in waterproof bags, carry a few basic survival items in your pockets. In the untoward event that your canoe tips over and you lose all your gear, you will still have those basic items—matches in a waterproof container, a signaling mirror, a whistle, a space blanket, a second copy of your map in a waterproof container, a compass, and a canoe repair kit.

Take good care of your life jackets; don't sit on them. When you step on shore for lunch or a walk, count the jackets to be sure they are all there. Then buckle them together and fasten them to the canoe. If one jacket were to drift away, it could be disastrous.

For you first canoe camping trip, consider going with others. Find an outdoors organization or a company that will include children in their trips and go with them. Look for these people in a canoeing magazine or through the state tourism office of the area you wish to visit.

Bicycle Touring

Cycle touring is a family activity that can include infants and toddlers. You often see cyclists taking their kids along, either in a little trailer behind the bike, on a seat behind the cyclist, or on a tandem bicycle; it all depends on the age of the child. In many ways, cycle touring is like backpacking or canoe camping, with all the family's clothing and other gear packed in panniers, those fat packs that fit over the back wheel of the bicycle.

Bicycle touring with children does not include rugged mountain biking. Of necessity, it is confined to roads or designated bicycle paths. The Rails-to-Trails movement has made it possible to convert many abandoned railroad rights-of-way to bicycle and/or hiking trails. Designed for railroad trains, the grade on these trails is generally quite gentle, often no more than 3 percent. In Wisconsin, in

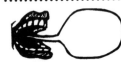

EXPERT'S ADVICE
Civilized Cycling

If you're looking for adventure close to civilization, consider bicycle touring. Cycling campers on roads or trails are close to cities and towns, so they can get along with carrying less food and other consumable supplies.

former stations in small towns along the trail, it is possible to rent bicycles and buy permits for the trail. Out-of-state residents pay more for the privilege of using the trails.

For information about Rails-to-Trails, write to Rails-to-Trails Conservancy, 1100 17th Street NW, Washington, DC 20036; call 202-331-9696; or find them on the web at www.railstrails.org. They publish a national directory of converted railroad beds.

Because they are riding so close to civilization, cyclists can get along with carrying less food and other supplies than backpacking or canoeing families. I was discussing diapers with a mom who has taken her kids on many trips. She told me that she uses disposable diapers and buys the smallest possible package at a time, because it's so easy to replenish the supply along the way. Same thing with food; it's a welcome change of pace for the group to stop along the way, shop for lunch, find a place to picnic, and let the kids run around and let off steam. It's especially good for toddlers who are more likely to get bored by the trip. They need frequent opportunities to get out of their seats.

Parks are good places to find water fountains to refill water bottles. Parents and kids should all drink lots of water. Sometimes adults who are peddling hard and carrying water in a backpack lose sight of the needs of their less active kids.

Infants in their trailers are usually content to ride, nap, or look at the scenery. Parents should fasten one or more tall flags to the trailer so that other traffic sees it. Check the child often to see that he or she is not too hot, too cold, too wet, thirsty, or otherwise unhappy. Even an infant likes to get out occasionally. Stop at a park, spread a tarp on the ground, and let the child kick and roll over.

Young children on the cycle with their parents should always wear properly fitting helmets. Even infants in their trailers should wear helmets, and, of course, parents should, too. Sometimes I see parents cycling with their children where the kids are wearing helmets but the parents are not. I shudder to think of the message that sends to the kids: helmets are for little kids, and grown-up people don't wear helmets.

Cycling families who have never bicycle camped should consider going with a group for the first time. Cycling organizations often plan trips that include a "sag wagon," a van that accompanies the group and picks up tired cyclists or their kids and drives them to the next campsite. You can find such trips on the web or in bicycling magazines.

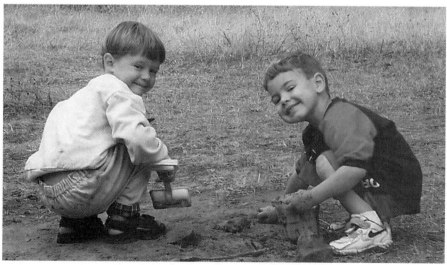

Any kind of camping is fun when you have a friend along.

Appendix: Resources

▶ Camping

▶ RVing

▶ Equipment

▶ Environmental Protection

▶ Safety Information

▶ Websites for Kids

▶ Information for Disabled Campers

Camping

Private Campgrounds

Kampgrounds of America: With 475 locations in the US and Canada, KOA is a very large organization of privately owned campgrounds that don't require a membership. Contact them at 406-248-7444 or www.koa.com.

Yogi Bear's Jellystone Camps: Most of these camps are in the eastern and southern states, with only a few as far west as Colorado and Montana. I love their website, which includes a special section, Just for Kids. Contact them at 800-558-2954 or www.campjellystone.com.

Western Horizon Resorts: Western Horizon has 22 camps in 13 states. While they are a membership organization, they often have promotional offers of three or four complimentary nights for potential members, and all you have to do is listen to a 90-minute presentation. Contact them at 866-453-9305 or www.whresorts.com.

Woodall's World of Travel: Woodall's publishes a number of different directories for campers, including the *North American Campground Directory* and *Go&Rent...Rent&Go*. They also publish a newsletter and organize RV tours. Contact them at 800-346-7572 or www.woodalls.com.

Public Parks

National Park Reservation Service: This service allows you to make campground reservations at some but not all national parks up to five months in advance. Contact at 800-365-2267 or reservations.nps.gov/index.cfm.

National Recreation Reservation Service: The NRRS offers reservation service for the US Forest Service, Army Corps of Engineers, National Park Service, Bureau of Land Management, and Bureau of Reclamation. Contact them at 877-444-6777 (TTY, 877-833-6777) or www.reserveusa.com.

Reserve America: This organization will make reservations at national parks and at some state and private campgrounds. They do not have a general phone number, but you can find phone numbers for the parks they serve at www.reserveamerica.com.

RVing

RV Rite: RV Rite provides a driver-training manual with fool-proof instructions for leveling procedures, proper water and sewer hook-ups, roadside emergencies and how to deal with them, and much, much more. Contact them at 253-435-8666 or www.rvrite.com.

RVers Online: This independent resource for RVers provides a bulletin board, RVing tips, and an advice service at www.rversonline.org.

GoRVing: This service was developed by RV dealers. They will send you a free "getting started" video for first-time RVers. Contact them at 703-620-6003 or www.gorving.com.

Good Sam Club: This organization of RV owners offers discounts and services for RV owners. Contact them at 800-234-3450 or www.goodsamclub.com.

Trailer Life: Contact this RV magazine at 800-825-6861 or www.trailerlife.com.

Motorhome: Contact this magazine at 800-678-1201 or www.motorhomemagazine.com.

Camping Life: Contact this magazine at 310-537-6322 or www.campinglife.com.

RV Life: Contact this magazine for the Northwest at 425-775-2911 or www.rvlife.com.

Renting RVs

Cruise America: Available in 40 states, this company offers "Fun Movers," units with a back wall that drops to allow a ramp for a wheelchair or all-terrain vehicle to slide out; they also have other RV models. Contact them at 800-671-8042 or www.cruiseamerica.com.

El Monte RV: This company offers RV rentals in California, Nevada, Florida, or New York. Contact them at 800-367-4808 or at www.elmonte.com.

Can Am Recreational Vehicles: This company has three rental outlets for motorhomes and travel trailers, in Winnipeg, Minnesota, and Washington state, but they sometimes deliver their RVs, once as far as Alaska. Contact them at 877-741-3860 or www.canamrv.com.

Equipment

General

REI: This national outdoor retail co-op has extensive rental departments. To find the branch nearest to you or for a catalog, call 800-426-4840 or go to www.rei.com.

Campmor: This New Jersey-based outdoor store offers the most extensive camping catalogue I know. Don't be fooled by the budget presentation; the quality of the goods is top notch. Contact them at 800-525-4784 or www.campmor.com.

Specialty Items

Coghlan's Camp Cooker: This is a the long-handled, cast-iron toasted sandwich maker or pie iron. Coghlan's is a manufacturer of camping equipment that wholesales to a number of retail outfits, including Home Town Stores, Ace Hardware, Global Market, and Amazon.com. Just search online for the Camp Cooker.

Happy Seat: This collapsed corrugated cardboard box opens to a toilet. It uses plastic bags inside that are biodegradable and can be tossed into an outhouse vault, meeting BLM and Forest Service regulations. Contact them at 970-878-4454 or www.happyseat.com.

Outback Pack: Outback Pack also offers a collapsed cardboard seat that has been tested for use by persons weighing up to 275 pounds. Contact them at 479-452-1893 or www.outbackpack.com.

Inflate-A-Potty: This blow-up plastic potty comes in two sizes, child and adult. Find out more online at www.potties.com.

Environmental Protection

Leave No Trace: This nonprofit education program promotes responsible outdoor recreation. Contact them at 800-332-4100 or www.lnt.org.

PEAK: This REI program promotes environmental awareness in kids. To find out more about the program, call 800-426-4840 or go to www.rei.com.

Insight Wildlife Management: This Washington-based organization seeks to nurture the role of humans as wildlife stewards through informed science and education. For more information, visit www.insightwildlife.com for a pamphlet on bears or write to PO Box 28656, Bellingham, Washington 98228.

Safety Information

Angel Alert Child Distance Monitor: This early-warning system detects when your child strays too far from adult supervision. Contact them at 800-706-7064, www.angelalert.net, or www.franzus.com.

Hug-A-Tree and Survive: This nationwide program, started by the San Diego Sheriff's Office Search and Rescue Unit, helps children learn what to do if they get lost. Contact them at 619-286-7536 or www.sdsheriff.net/SAR/pr/hugatree.html.

Stay Put, Stay Dry: This program of the outdoor retail shop Eastern Mountain Sports is also aimed at helping children know what to do if they get lost. Visit www.ems.com and click on Store Locations to find a shop near you.

First Aid

Mountaineering Medicine: This book, by Fred T. Darvill, Jr. M.D., is also published by Wilderness Press (1998).

Backcountry First Aid and Extended Care: This book, by Buck Tilton, is published by Falcon (2002).

American Red Cross First Aid & Safety Handbook: This book, by Kathleen A. Handal, is published by Little Brown (1992).

Websites For Kids

www.50states.com: Provides all sorts of information about the states.

www.nps.gov: The National Park Service site offers kids an opportunity to learn about national parks, monuments, seashores, historical sites, and forests. Click on Interpretation and Education, then click on GoZONE.

www.nps.gov/learn/juniorranger.html: Learn about the National Park Service's Junior Ranger Programs.

www.nps.gov/webrangers: Learn about the National Park Service's WebRanger program.

www.stardate.org: The site, administered by the University of Texas McDonald Observatory, offers information about the stars and the planets.

www.famboomerang.com: Learn about "Seeker," a scavenger hunt game.

Information for Disabled Campers

Easter Seals Society: This national organization has chapters all over the country that offer information and equipment to the disabled. Contact them at 800-221-6827 or www.easterseals.org.

National Center on Physical Activity and Disability: This is an informational resource to agencies all over the country that offer programs and equipment to the disabled. Contact them at 800-900-8086 or www.ncpad.org.

Disabled Sports USA: This is another clearinghouse for agencies all over the country that offer the disabled programs and equipment. Contact them at 301-217-0960 or www.dsusa.org.

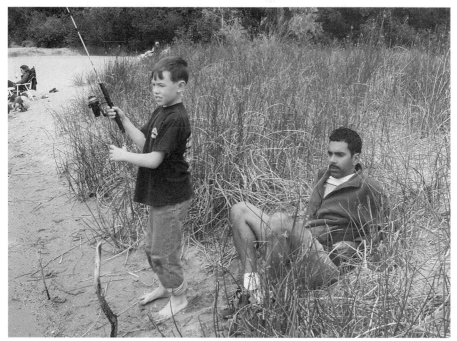

Father and son bond while waiting for the big one.

Index

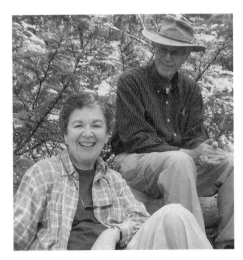

About the Author

Goldie Gendler Silverman (pictured here with her husband, Don) grew up in Nebraska and learned to camp in Washington, Oregon, California, Idaho, and Arizona. After several years of teaching English at the high school and university levels, she began writing remedial reading textbooks, co-authored four cookbooks, and then went on to write *Backpacking with Babies and Small Children*, published first by Signpost Books and later by Wilderness Press. Mother of three grown children and two almost-grown grandchildren, Goldie now hikes all over the world, but still backpacks with her family near her home in Seattle.

Photo Credits

Henk Dawson, Jr.: ii, 2, 22, 33, 34, 41, 44, 48, 54, 60, 65, 69, 74, 80, 82, 109, 110, 113, 114, 125, 133, 143, 164, 168, 174, 190

Jon Ostrow: ix, 16, 20, 73, 85, 117, 167, 172, 177, 181, 186, 197, 201, 216, 236

Don Silverman: x, 9, 13, 25, 27, 28, 31, 37, 51, 77, 90, 95, 99, 105, 120, 125, 128, 134, 138, 146, 149, 152, 159, 210, 226, 230

Goldie Gendler Silverman: 56

Sarah Silverman: 154, 156, 163